Clinicians' Guides to Radionuclide Hybrid Imaging

PET/CT

Series Editors

Jamshed B. Bomanji
London, UK

Gopinath Gnanasegaran
London, UK

Stefano Fanti
Bologna, Italy

Homer A. Macapinlac
Houston, Texas, USA

Hybrid imaging with PET/CT and SPECT/CT provides high-quality information on function and structure, thereby permitting accurate localization, characterization, and diagnosis. There is extensive evidence to support the value of PET/CT, which has made a significant impact on oncological imaging and the management of patients with cancer. The evidence in favor of SPECT/CT, especially for orthopaedic indications, is evolving and increasing. This pocket book series on hybrid imaging (PET/CT and SPECT/CT) is specifically aimed at referring clinicians, nuclear medicine/radiology physicians, radiographers/technologists, and nurses who routinely work in nuclear medicine and participate in multidisciplinary meetings. The series will include 18 pocket books on PET/CT and 3 on SPECT/CT. Compiled under the auspices of the British Nuclear Medicine Society, the series is the joint work of many colleagues and professionals worldwide who share a common vision and purpose in promoting and supporting nuclear medicine as an important imaging specialty for the diagnosis and management of oncological and non-oncological conditions.

The PET/CT pocket book series will be dedicated to some of the Society's recently departed peers, including Prof Ignac Fogelman, Dr Muriel Buxton-Thomas and Prof Ajit K Padhy.

More information about this series at http://www.springer.com/series/13803

Archi Agrawal · Venkatesh Rangarajan
Ameya D. Puranik
Editors

PET/CT in Non-Hodgkin Lymphoma

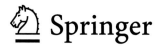 Springer

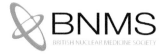

Editors
Archi Agrawal
Nuclear Medicine and Molecular Imaging
Tata Memorial Hospital
Mumbai, Maharashtra
India

Venkatesh Rangarajan
Nuclear Medicine and Molecular Imaging
Tata Memorial Hospital
Mumbai, Maharashtra
India

Ameya D. Puranik
Nuclear Medicine and Molecular Imaging
Tata Memorial Hospital
Mumbai, Maharashtra
India

ISSN 2367-2439   ISSN 2367-2447 (electronic)
Clinicians' Guides to Radionuclide Hybrid Imaging - PET/CT
ISBN 978-3-030-79006-6   ISBN 978-3-030-79007-3   (eBook)
https://doi.org/10.1007/978-3-030-79007-3

This Springer imprint is published by the registered company Springer Nature Switzerland AG
The registered company address is: Gewerbestrasse 11, 6330 Cham, Switzerland

PET/CT series is dedicated to Prof. Ignac Fogelman, Dr. Muriel Buxton-Thomas and Prof. Ajit K. Padhy.

Foreword

Clear and concise clinical indications for PET/CT in the management of the oncology patient are presented in this series of 20 separate booklets. The impact on better staging, tailored management and specific treatment of the patient with cancer has been achieved with the advent of this multimodality imaging technology. Early and accurate diagnosis will always pay, and clear information can be gathered with PET/CT on treatment responses. Prognostic information is gathered and can forward guide additional therapeutic options.

It is a fortunate coincidence that PET/CT was able to derive great benefit from radionuclide-labelled probes, which deliver good and often excellent target to non-target signals. Whilst labelled glucose remains the cornerstone for the clinical benefit achieved, a number of recent probes are definitely adding benefit. PET/CT is hence an evolving technology, extending its applications and indications. Significant advances in the instrumentation and data processing available have also contributed to this technology, which delivers high throughput and a wealth of data, with good patient tolerance and indeed patient and public acceptance. As an example, the role of PET/CT in the evaluation of cardiac disease is also covered, with an emphasis on labelled rubidium and labelled glucose studies.

The novel probes of labelled choline, labelled peptides, such as DOTATATE, and, most recently, labelled PSMA (prostate-specific membrane antigen) have gained rapid clinical utility and acceptance, as significant PET/CT tools for the management of neuroendocrine disease and prostate cancer patients, notwithstanding all the advances achieved with other imaging modalities, such as MRI. Hence, a chapter reviewing novel PET tracers forms part of this series.

The oncological community has recognised the value of PET/CT and has delivered advanced diagnostic criteria for some of the most important indications for PET/CT. This includes the recent Deauville criteria for the classification of PET/CT patients with lymphoma—similar criteria are expected to develop for other malignancies, such as head and neck cancer, melanoma and pelvic malignancies. For completion, a separate section covers the role of PET/CT in radiotherapy planning, discussing the indications for planning biological tumour volumes in relevant cancers.

These booklets offer simple, rapid and concise guidelines on the utility of PET/CT in a range of oncological indications. They also deliver a rapid aide memoire on the merits and appropriate indications for PET/CT in oncology.

London, UK   Peter J. Ell, FMedSci, DR HC, AΩA

Preface

The *Hybrid Imaging* with PET/CT and SPECT/CT combines best of function and structure to provide accurate localisation, characterisation and diagnosis. There is extensive literature and evidence to support PET/CT, which has made significant impact in oncological imaging and management of patients with cancer. The evidence in favour of SPECT/CT especially in orthopaedic indications is evolving and increasing.

The *Hybrid Imaging* (PET/CT and SPECT/CT) pocketbook series is specifically aimed at our referring clinicians, nuclear medicine/radiology doctors, radiographers/technologists and nurses who are routinely working in nuclear medicine and participate in Multi-Disciplinary Meetings. This series is the joint work of many friends and professionals from different nations who share a common dream and vision towards promoting and supporting nuclear medicine as a useful and important imaging speciality.

We want to thank all those people who have contributed to this work as advisors, authors and reviewers, without whom the book would not have been possible. We want to thank our members from the BNMS (British Nuclear Medicine Society, UK) for their encouragement and support, and we are extremely grateful to Dr. Brian Nielly, Charlotte Weston, the BNMS Education Committee and the BNMS council members for their enthusiasm and trust.

Finally, we wish to extend particular gratitude to the industry for their continuous support towards education and training.

London, UK   Gopinath Gnanasegaran
London, UK   Jamshed B. Bomanji

Acknowledgements

The series co-ordinators and editors would like to express sincere gratitude to the members of the British Nuclear Medicine Society, patients, teachers, colleagues, students, the industry and the BNMS Education Committee Members for their continued support and inspiration.

Andy Bradley
Brent Drake
Francis Sundram
James Ballinger
Parthiban Arumugam
Rizwan Syed
Sai Han
Vineet Prakash

Contents

List of Contributors and Editors

Series Editors

Jamshed Bomanji, MBBS, MSc, PhD, FRCP, FRCR Department of Nuclear Medicine, University College London Hospitals NHS Foundation Trust, London, UK

Gopinath Gnanasegaran, MBBS, MSc, MD, FRCP Royal Free London NHS Foundation Trust, London, UK

Stefano Fanti, MD University of Bologna, Bologna, Italy

Nuclear Medicine Division and PET Unit at the Policlinico S.Orsola, University of Bologna, Bologna, Italy

Specialty School of Nuclear Medicine at University of Bologna, Bologna, Italy

Homer Macapinlac, MD Division of Diagnostic Imaging, Department of Nuclear Medicine, The University of Texas MD Anderson Cancer Center, Houston, TX, USA

Editors

Archi Agrawal, DMRE, DRM, DNB Department of Nuclear Medicine and Molecular Imaging, Tata Memorial Hospital, Homi Bhabha National Institute, Mumbai, India

Ameya D. Puranik, DNB, FEBNM Department of Nuclear Medicine and Molecular Imaging, Tata Memorial Hospital, Homi Bhabha National Institute, Mumbai, India

Venkatesh Rangarajan, DRM, DNB Department of Nuclear Medicine and Molecular Imaging, Tata Memorial Hospital, Homi Bhabha National Institute, Mumbai, India

Contributors

Hasmukh Jain, DM Medical Oncology, Tata Memorial Hospital, Homi Bhabha National Institute, Mumbai, India

Abhinav Zawar, DM Medical Oncology, Tata Memorial Hospital, Homi Bhabha National Institute, Mumbai, India

Jayashree Thorat Tata Memorial Hospital, Homi Bhabha National Institute, Mumbai, India

Sridhar Epari Department of Pathology, Tata Memorial Hospital and ACTREC, Homi Bhabha National Institute, Mumbai, India

Vasu Babu Goli Department of Medical Oncology, Tata Memorial Hospital, Homi Bhabha National Institute, Mumbai, India

Manju Sengar Department of Medical Oncology, Tata Memorial Hospital, Homi Bhabha National Institute, Mumbai, India

Nilendu C. Purandare Department of Nuclear Medicine, Tata Memorial Hospital, Homi Bhabha National Institute, Mumbai, India

Suman Kumar Ankathi Department of Radiology, Tata Memorial Hospital, Homi Bhabha National Institute, Mumbai, India

Archi Agrawal, DRM, DNB Department of Nuclear Medicine and Molecular Imaging, Tata Memorial Hospital, Homi Bhabha National Institute, Mumbai, India

M. V. Manikandan, MD Department of Nuclear Medicine and Molecular Imaging, Tata Memorial Hospital, Homi Bhabha National Institute, Mumbai, India

Abhishek Uppal, MD Department of Nuclear Medicine and Molecular Imaging, Tata Memorial Hospital, Homi Bhabha National Institute, Mumbai, India

Venkatesh Rangarajan, DRM, DNB Department of Nuclear Medicine and Molecular Imaging, Tata Memorial Hospital, Homi Bhabha National Institute, Mumbai, India

Ameya D. Puranik Department of Nuclear Medicine and Molecular Imaging, Tata Memorial Hospital, Homi Bhabha National Institute, Mumbai, India

Sneha Shah Department of Nuclear Medicine and Molecular Imaging, Tata Memorial Hospital, Homi Bhabha National Institute, Mumbai, India

Sayak Choudhury Department of Nuclear Medicine and Molecular Imaging, Tata Memorial Centre Advanced Centre for Treatment, Research and Education in Cancer, Homi Bhabha National Institute, Mumbai, India

Introduction to Non-Hodgkin's Lymphoma

1

Hasmukh Jain, Abhinav Zawar, and Jayashree Thorat

Contents

1.1 Non-Hodgkin's Lymphoma

Non-Hodgkin's Lymphoma (NHL) arises from the lymphoid system and is grouped as B and T cell lymphomas. They represent 4% of all the cancers in USA [1].

H. Jain (✉) · A. Zawar · J. Thorat
Department of Medical Oncology, Tata Memorial Hospital, Homi Bhabha National Institute, Mumbai, India

© The Author(s), under exclusive license to Springer Nature Switzerland AG 2021
A. Agrawal et al. (eds.), *PET/CT in Non-Hodgkin Lymphoma*, Clinicians' Guides to Radionuclide Hybrid Imaging, https://doi.org/10.1007/978-3-030-79007-3_1

1

1.1.1 Biology of Lymphomas

Lymphomas originate from the lymphocytes at various stages of their development (Table 1.1).

1.1.2 Risk Factors

In more than 90%, the exact cause is unknown. However, in a small subset a specific etiology can be identified (Table 1.2).

The specific diagnosis can be suspected based on

1. The extent of adenopathy, i.e., localized or generalized.
2. Presentation (Table 1.3).

1.1.3 WHO Classification of NHL: (Table 1.4)

1.1.3.1 Clinical Features in NHL

The clinical course can be indolent or aggressive depending on the subtype. Early bone marrow involvement, extra-axial nodes, and extra nodal sites with noncontiguous dissemination characterize NHL. Majority of them present with painless adenopathy and

Table 1.1 The classification of B- and T-cell lymphoma according to the cell of origin

B cell	Normal counterpart	Disease
Bone marrow	Progenitor B cell	B lymphoblastic leukemia/lymphoma
	Precursor B cell	
	Immature B cell	
Lymph node	Naïve B cell	CLL/SLL
	Pre-germinal center	Mantle cell lymphoma
	Germinal center B cell	Follicular lymphoma, Burkitt's lymphoma, DLBCL, Hodgkin's lymphoma
	Marginal zone B cell	Marginal zone and MALT lymphoma Lymphoplasmacytic lymphoma CLL/SLL (some)
	Plasma cell	Plasma cell myeloma
T cell	Precursor cell	Disease
Thymus	Double negative T cells (No CD4/8 and non-rearranged T cell receptor-TCR)	T lymphoblastic leukemia/lymphoma
	Double positive (CD4, 8 and express complete TCR)	
Lymph node	TH1 cells	Peripheral T-cell lymphoma NOS (subset)
	TH2 cells	Subset of PTCL, NOS
	Follicular helper T cells	Angioimmunoblastic T-cell lymphoma PTCL-FHT cell type
	Regulatory T cells	Adult-T cell leukemia/lymphoma

Table 1.2 Risk factors associated with lymphoma

Viral infection	
EBV	Burkitt's lymphoma, Post-transplant lymphoproliferative disorder
HTLV-1	Adult T-cell leukemia/lymphoma
HHV-8	Kaposi sarcoma, Primary effusion lymphoma
Hepatitis C virus	Splenic marginal zone lymphoma
Hepatitis B virus	Diffuse large B- cell lymphoma
Bacterial infection	
Helicobacter pylori	Gastric Maltoma
Chlamydia psittaci	Orbital Maltoma
Borrelia burgdorferi/afzeliﬁ	Cutaneous Maltoma
Campylobacter jejuni	Immunoproliferative small intestinal disease
Primary immunodeficiency	
Ataxia-telangiectasia	Both B & T Cell NHL
Wiskott-Aldrich syndrome	DLBCL, NHL of larynx
X-linked lymphoproliferative syndrome	NHL
Severe combined immunodeficiency	NHL, HL, EBV associated Burkitt's lymphoma
Acquired conditions of immunodeficiency	
HIV infections	DLBCL, Burkitt's Ƚlymphoma, primary CNS Ƚlymphoma, Plasmablastic lymphoma, primary effusion lymphoma
Organ or stem cell transplantation	Post-transplant lymphoproliferative disorder(PTLD)
Autoimmune and rheumatologic disease	
Rheumatoid arthritis	Hodgkin's lymphoma, PTCL, TLGL
Systemic lupus erythematosus	DLBCL
Sjögren's syndrome	Marginal zone lymphoma, Lymphoplasmacytic lymphoma, DLBCL
Celiac disease	Intestinal T- cell lymphoma
Hashimoto's thyroiditis	Follicular center cell lymphoma
Environmental or occupational	
Herbicides/pesticides	Non- Hodgkin's lymphoma
Anti TNF	B cell NHL, Hepatosplenic γδ T lymphoma
Phenytoin/carbamazepine	Pseudo lymphoma and malignant lymphoma
Breast implant associated	ALCL

extra nodal involvement can be detected in up to 40%. Systemic symptoms occur in approximately 25%. Cytopenias (rare) occur due to marrow involvement, immune mediated, hypersplenism, or hemophagocytic lymphohistiocytosis.

1.1.3.2 Workup for NHL (Table 1.5)

PET using 18-Fluorodeoxyglucose is used to stage and assess response to therapy. It improves accuracy of staging for both nodal and extra nodal compared to CT scan leading to change in stage in 10–30%. Interim PET scan positivity has shown inferior outcome in Hodgkin's lymphoma [3] but failed to predict outcome in DLBCL [4, 5]. 18-FDG uptake varies according to histology and proliferative activity with less uptake in indolent lymphoma than aggressive.

Table 1.3 Differential diagnosis based on pattern of presentation and extra nodal site of involvement

A. Based on pattern of presentation

Presentation	Aggressive	Indolent
Extent		
Localized	DLBCL	HL/NLPHL
	Burkitt's lymphoma	Follicular lymphoma
	ALCL	Nodal MZL
Generalized	DLBCL	CLL
	Lymphoblastic lymphoma	FL
	PTCL	Splenic MZL
	ALCL	Hairy cell leukemia
	Mantle cell lymphoma	Lymphoplasmacytic lymphoma
	Follicular lymphoma grade III	Mycosis Fungoides
		T-cell LGL

B. Based on extra nodal site involvement

Sl. No	Site	Entities
1.	Skin	Primary cutaneous lymphoma
		ALCL
		AITL
		ATLL
		T-PLL
2.	CNS	DLBCL
		BL
		Dural marginal zone lymphoma
		LPL—Bing–Neel syndrome
		T-cell lymphoma- ATLL,T-PLL
3.	GIT	DLBCL
		Burkitt's lymphoma
		Mantle cell lymphoma
		Maltoma
		Follicular lymphoma
		EATL
		Heavy chain disease
4.	Splenomegaly predominant	Mantle cell lymphoma
		SMZL
		Hairy cell leukemia
		T-PLL
		Lymphoplasmacytic lymphoma
		HSTL
		HCL variant
		Follicular lymphoma
5.	Ocular and extra ocular	DLBCL
		PCNSL
		Maltoma
6.	AIHA	CLL/SLL
		Follicular lymphoma
		AITL

Table 1.4   WHO classification of NHL [2]

Mature B cell neoplasms	Mature T cell neoplasms
Aggressive neoplasms	**Leukemic or disseminated**
Diffuse large B-cell lymphoma: Variants, subgroups, and subtypes	T-cell large granular lymphocytic leukemia
Diffuse large B-cell lymphoma (DLBCL), NOS	Chronic lymphoproliferative
Germinal center B-cell type	disorders of NK cells T-cell
Activated B-cell type	T-cell prolymphocytic leukemia
	Aggressive NK-cell leukemia
	Adult T-cell leukemia/lymphoma
Diffuse large B-cell lymphoma subtypes	**Extra nodal**
T-cell/ histiocyte-rich large B-cell lymphoma	Extra nodal NK/T-cell lymphoma, nasal type
Primary DLBCL of the CNS	Enteropathy-type T-cell lymphoma
Primary cutaneous DLBCL, leg type	Hepatosplenic T-cell lymphoma
DLBCL associated with chronic inflammation	Breast implant-associated
HHV8-positive DLBCL, NOS	anaplastic large-cell lymphoma
EBV-positive DLBCL, NOS	**Cutaneous**
Other lymphomas of large B cells	Mycosis fungoides
Primary mediastinal large B-cell lymphoma	Sezary syndrome
Intravascular large B-cell lymphoma	Primary cutaneous anaplastic
EBV-positive mucocutaneous ulcer	large-cell lymphoma
ALK-positive large B-cell lymphoma	Lymphomatoid papulosis
Plasmablastic lymphoma	Subcutaneous panniculitis-like
Multicentric Castleman disease	T-cell lymphoma
Primary effusion lymphoma	Primary cutaneous $\gamma\delta$ T-cell lymphoma
	Nodal
B-cell lymphoma, unclassifiable, with features intermediate between DLBCL and classical Hodgkin lymphoma	Peripheral T-cell lymphoma (PTCL), NOS
	Angioimmunoblastic T-cell lymphoma (AITL)
	Follicular T-cell lymphoma
	Nodal peripheral T-cell lymphoma with TFH phenotype
	Anaplastic large-cell lymphoma (ALCL), ALK positive
	Anaplastic large-cell lymphoma, ALK negative
High-grade B-cell lymphoma, with MYC and BCL2 and/ or BCL6 rearrangements	
High-grade B-cell lymphoma, NOS	
Burkitt's lymphoma	
Mantle cell lymphoma	
Indolent lymphomas	

(continued)

Table 1.4 (continued)

Mature B cell neoplasms	Mature T cell neoplasms
Follicular lymphoma	
Extra nodal marginal zone lymphoma of mucosa-associated lymphoid tissue (MALT)	
Nodal marginal zone lymphoma	
Splenic marginal zone lymphoma	
Lymphoplasmacytic lymphoma	
Heavy chain disease	
Plasma cell neoplasms	
CLL/SLL	
Monoclonal B-cell lymphocytosis	
B-cell prolymphocytic leukemia (PLL)	
Hairy cell leukemia	

Table 1.5 Staging work up

Staging workup for lymphoma
Initial studies
History and physical examination (including B symptoms, any immunosuppression, autoimmune disease, HIV)
Complete blood count with peripheral smear examination
Biochemistry—Renal function with uric acid and liver function tests
Lactate dehydrogenase and/ or $\beta_2$microglobulin
Hepatitis B, C and HIV Serologies
Tumor biopsy preferably excisional with histopathology
Site preferred for biopsy—cervical > axillary > inguinal
Immunohistochemistry of tumor specimen
Cytogenetic analysis of tumor specimen (if lymphoma associated translocations suspected)
PET/CT scans for FDG avid lymphomas
Contrast enhanced CT scan of neck, chest, abdomen, and pelvis (FDG non-avid lymphomas)
Cardiac ejection fraction measurement (anthracycline based therapy)
Pregnancy testing in women of child bearing age
Additional studies in selected cases
Bone marrow study with aspiration and biopsy
Lumbar puncture with cytology and flow cytometry
Magnetic resonance imaging of brain if neurologic signs or symptoms
Immunoglobulin and TCR gene rearrangement studies

18-FDG PET scan can be used for staging in FDG-avid lymphomas such as DLBCL, Hodgkin's lymphoma, Follicular lymphoma whereas in non-FDG avid lymphomas, a contrast-enhanced CT scan is preferred.

The current staging system for NHL in adults is the **Lugano classification** [6]. Stage I involves one node or a group of adjacent nodes or single extra nodal lesion without nodal involvement. Stage II involves two or more lymph node regions on the same side of the diaphragm or Stage II by nodal extent with limited contiguous extra nodal extension. Limited stage (I or II) lymphomas that affect an organ outside the lymph system (an extra nodal organ) have an E added (for example, stage IIE). Stage III is involvement of lymph node regions on both sides of the diaphragm, nodes above the diaphragm with or spleen involvement. Stage IV is widely spread into at least one organ outside the lymph system, such as the bone marrow, liver, or lung.

1.1.4   Prognostic Indices (Table 1.6)

The International prognostic index (IPI) applies for untreated aggressive NHL with 1 point assigned to each factor and score of 1, 2, 3, and 4 to 5 correspond to 5 year survival of 73%, 51%, 43%, and 26%, respectively, in the pre-rituximab era [7]. The Revised IPI(R-IPI) was developed to predict the outcome of individuals receiving rituximab with chemotherapy [8].

Table 1.6 Prognostic indices

R-IPI (1 point each)	NCCN IPI (1 point each)	FLIPI (1 point each)	MIPI (Simplified)
Age > 60 years	Age 41–60 years—1 point	Age > 60 years	Age < 50 years—0 point
	Age > 60–75 years—2 point		Age 50–59 years—1point
	Age > 75 years—3 point		Age 60–69 years—2 point
			Age ≥ 70 years—3 point
Performance status ≥2	Performance status ≥2—1 point	Hemoglobin <12 g/L	Performance status 0–1—0 point
			Performance status 2–4—2 point
LDH above normal	LDH ratio 1–3—1 point	LDH above normal	LDH:ULN ratio <0.67—0 point
			0.67–0.99—1 point
	LDH ratio > 3—2 point		1.00–1.49—2 point
			≥1.50—3 point
Ann Arbor stage III or IV	Ann Arbor stage III or IV	Stage III or IV	Leucocyte count (10⁹/L) <6.7—0 point
			06.7–9.9—1 point
			10.0–14.9—2 point
			≥15.0—3 point
Number of extra nodal sites >1	Extra nodal disease involving the bone marrow, central nervous system, liver/gastrointestinal tract, or lung – 1 point	Number of nodal sites >4	
Risk group—3 year OS	Risk group—5 year OS	Risk group—2 year OS	Risk group—5 year OS
0–1—91	0–1—96	0–1—98	0–3—60
2—81	2–3—77	2—94	4–5—35
3—65	4–5—56	≥3—87	6–12—20
4–5—59	>5—35		

The National Comprehensive Cancer Network (NCCN)-IPI incorporates detailed information about the clinical variables used in the original IPI [9]. The Follicular Lymphoma International Prognostic Index (FLIPI) and Mantle Cell Lymphoma International Prognostic Index (MIPI) have been found to reliably predict survival in follicular lymphoma [10] and mantle cell lymphoma [11].

1.1.5 Specific Features of Common Subtypes

1.1.5.1 Follicular Lymphoma

Epidemiology and pathology: The most common indolent lymphoma with a median age of presentation of 64 years, and a female predominance [12]. FLs are derived from germinal center B cell and graded based on centroblasts per high power field: Grade 1–2 (0–15), Grade 3 A(>15) centroblasts present and 3B with sheets of centroblasts [13].

Clinical features: Asymptomatic lymphadenopathy, extra nodal disease is less common, B symptoms present in 20% cases and bone marrow involvement seen in 70% cases.

Immunophenotype: FL cells express CD 10, CD 20, and BCL-6 and anti-apoptotic protein BCL 2. The overexpression of anti-apoptotic BCL2 is mediated by t (14:18) which juxtaposes BCL2 gene to the Ig heavy chain locus in 85% cases.

Evaluation: PET/CT scan is particularly useful to stage or to identify the site for biopsy in suspected transformed disease.

1.1.5.2 DLBCL

Epidemiology: Most common NHL subtype [2] with median age of 65 years and male predominance.

Clinical features: Nodal or extra nodal disease and bone marrow involvement in fewer than 10% cases.

Immunophenotype: B cell markers CD 19, 20, 22 & 79a and germinal B cell markers include CD 10, BCL6. CD5 and BCL2 are variable positive. Rearrangements in the MYC oncogene are found in ~15% of DLBCL and are associated with BCL2 or BCL6 and termed as "double hit" lymphomas or "triple hit" when all three are present.

Evaluation: Bone marrow biopsy is not recommended if bone marrow involvement is indicated by PET and if imaging is negative it is appropriate to consider biopsy. CSF analysis is to be considered with clinical features of CNS disease, high CNS IPI (4–6), 2 or more extra nodal disease sites irrespective of CNS IPI and testicular, renal/adrenal or intravascular involvement, double hit/triple hit lymphoma.

1.1.5.3 Specific Clinicopathologic Entities of DLBCL

Primary mediastinal(thymic) large B-cell Lymphoma—Both clinically and biologically more closely resemble classical HL, with median age of presentation of 35 years and female preponderance [14].

T-cell/ histiocyte–rich large B-cell lymphoma—Uncommon variant (<10%) of DLBCL; mainly in middle-aged males [15].

1.1.6 Primary CNS Lymphoma

Epidemiology: 1% of all NHL, with median age of 65 years and male predominance. Risk factors include immunosuppression, HIV infection, and autoimmune disease.

Clinical features: Neurocognitive symptoms are most common, focal neurodeficits as per site are common presentation.

Immunophenotype: B cell markers CD 19, 20, 22 positive, BCL2 variable, BCL 6 + (50%), CD 10 negative. 95% of PCNSLs are DLBCL [16].

Evaluation: CSF, bone marrow studies, and contrast enhanced MRI Brain & systemic imaging to determine disease extent. Slit lamp examination and stereotactic needle biopsy of brain are indicated in most of cases. Prognostication done using IELSG score (age, PS, LDH, deep seated brain tumors, and elevated CSF proteins) [17].

1.1.7 Marginal Zone Lymphoma

Epidemiology and pathology: Indolent neoplasm of mature post-germinal center B lymphocytes [18]. About 10% of all NHL with three subtypes nodal, extra nodal, and splenic MZL.

MZL arise with chronic antigenic stimulation due to pathogens or autoimmune diseases; or translocations result in Ag independent activation of NF-kB.

Clinical features: They vary as per the site of involvement, for example, lymphadenopathy (Nodal MZL), orbital mass, parotid mass, cough (bronchial MZL), skin nodules (Cutaneous MALT), epigastric pain (Gastric MALT), intestinal obstruction (SI), splenomegaly (splenic MZL), and B symptoms.

Immunophenotype: Cell markers CD19, 20, 22; CD 5, 10, cyclin D1 negative.

Cytogenetics [19]: Most common is t(11;18), other t(1;14), t(14;18).

Evaluation: Baseline evaluation as suggested above with SPEP (paraprotein often present) should be considered. BM aspirate and biopsy in splenic MZL show intrasinusoidal lymphocytic infiltration. Upper GI endoscopy in Gastric MALT for biopsy and H. pylori testing.

Imaging with Contrast CT Chest/abdomen/pelvis; MRI orbits (Ocular MALT). FDG PET scan not considered.

1.1.8 Mantle Cell Lymphoma

Epidemiology and pathology: 6% of all NHL with male predominance and median age of 70 years.

Clinical features: Clinical behavior is intermediate between indolent and aggressive with strong tendency to present in advanced stage. Lymphadenopathy with extra nodal involvement is common including bone marrow involvement.

Immunophenotype: CD 19, 20 (B cell markers), CD5 (aberrant expression of T cell) but negative for CD200/23 (CLL) or CD 10(FL).

Cytogenetics: t(11; 14) which juxtaposes cyclin D1 with Ig heavy chain locus is the hallmark (overexpression of cyclinD1).

Evaluation: Peripheral blood flow/bone marrow biopsy as leukemic phase disease is common, and pan-endoscopy as GI tract is commonly involved. Ki67 (>30% or <30%), p53 abnormality, and SOX 11 expression are prognostic factors and predict for aggressive disease.

1.1.9 Burkitt's Lymphoma

Among the most aggressive of all human malignancies with acute onset, rapid doubling time <24 h, and B symptoms.

Epidemiology and pathology: Arise from germinal center B cell, with translocations that dysregulate MYC expression by placing it under control of Ig gene enhancer. Histology shows monotonous sheet of medium sized atypical B cells, extensive necrosis, frequent mitosis (Ki67 95%), and classic starry sky pattern (Sky—Burkitt's cells with lipid droplets and starry—macrophages with apoptotic debris within).

Distinct clinical forms:

Endemic—In equatorial Africa with strong association for EBV, male predominance and commonly presents as jaw mass.

Sporadic—30% of pediatric lymphoma and <1% of adult NHL with peak age 11 years and 30 years, respectively. Commonly extra nodal presentation as abdominal lump.

Immunodeficiency associated—In HIV positive & EBV negative, CD4 independent, HAART has no impact on incidence and usually present in adult with both nodal and extra nodal disease.

Immunophenotype: CD19, 20, 22 positive (B cell markers), CD 10 & Bcl-6 positive (germinal center).

Characterized by MYC translocation t(8;14) in 85% cases or t(2;8) or t(8;22).

Evaluation: Bone marrow study and lumbar puncture to rule out CNS involvement. Imaging with contrast enhanced thorax, abdomen, and pelvis to determine disease extent.

1.1.10 Hairy Cell Leukemia

Epidemiology and pathology: 2% of all leukemia with median age of presentation of 50 years and male predominance.

Clinical features: Constitutional symptoms with massive splenomegaly and symptomatic cytopenias. *Immunophenotype*: Mature B cell markers present are CD19, 20, 22 with CD25; aberrant expression of CD 11c, CD103, CD123.

Evaluation: Peripheral smear shows small–medium size mononuclear cells with finger like projections (hairy cells), BM biopsy is hypercellular within filtrating hairy cells; abundant cytoplasm surrounding the nuclei give the appearance of fried egg. Often the bone marrow aspirate is dry tap.

1.1.11 Peripheral T-Cell Lymphoma

10% of all NHL, male predominance and median age of 65 years.

Aggressive neoplasms arising from mature T lymphocytes and NK Cells with poor response to chemotherapy and OS relative to B cell, exception ALCL, skin limited mycosis fungoides have excellent prognosis. Presentation is prominent B symptoms with pruritus, generalized lymphadenopathy, hepatosplenomegaly; extra nodal disease and 70% have advanced disease.

Investigations: Baseline NHL workup and other tests to be considered are coombs test (if AIHA suspected), HTLV 1 serology (ATLL), Serum EBV PCR (NK/T-cell Lymphoma). Imaging with PET CT scan for disease extent.

1.1.11.1 Types
PTCL NOS: MC subtype of PTCLs, accounting for 30% of cases.

AITL (Angioimmunoblastic T-Cell Lymphoma): Account for 15–20% of cases with median age of 65 years.

ALCL (Anaplastic Large-Cell Lymphoma): CD 30 positive subtype of PTCL with two biologically distinct diseases; ALK positive ALCL that overexpresses ALK due to t(2;5) and ALK negative ALCL.

ALK positive usually present in young age group and has better prognosis compared to ALK negative ALCL.

Primary cutaneous ALCL: Indolent behavior, predominant dermatologic involvement. Second most common type of CTCL with median age of presentation is 60 years but favorable outcomes.

Breast implant associated ALCL: ALCL associated with implants (silicone and saline) with CD30 + and ALK negative. Typical localized presentation with unexplained seroma or capsular thickening.

Extra nodal NK/T-cell lymphoma: Mainly seen in Asian males aged 40–50 years and associated with EBV. Typically involves midline sinus/palate but involvement of other sites can occur.

ATLL (Adult T-Cell Lymphoma & Leukemia): Endemic in Southwestern Japan, Caribbean basin where HTLV-1 prevalence is high. There are four clinical variants: Acute, lymphoma type, chronic, and smoldering. The most common is the acute form with elevated white blood count, skin rash, lymphadenopathy, hepatosplenomegaly, pulmonary infiltrates, and hypercalcemia with or without lytic bone lesions.

1.1.12 Cutaneous T-Cell Lymphoma (CTCL)

5% of NHL with primary involvement of skin.

1.1.12.1 Types

Mycosis fungoides (MF): Most common CTCL (50%) with indolent clinical course and primary involvement of skin. In early stage appears as plaques or patches with pruritus and gradually evolves to diffuse erythroderma or tumor usually associated with adenopathy. Extra cutaneous involvement occurs in advanced stage of disease with histologic transformation.

Sezary Syndrome (SS): Characterized by erythroderma, generalized lymphadenopathy, presence of Sezary cells in skin, lymph nodes, and peripheral blood.

1.2 Summary and Conclusions

Non-Hodgkin lymphomas encompass several subtypes with unique clinical, biological characteristics. A multidisciplinary approach is essential for correct diagnosis, staging, and management.

Acknowledgement Dr. Krishna Prasad for simplifying the concepts of lymphoma.

References

1. Lymphoma—Non-Hodgkin: Statistics|Cancer.Net.   https://www.cancer.net/cancer-types/lymphoma-non-hodgkin/statistics. Accessed 22 Nov 2020.
2. Swerdlow SH, Campo E, Pileri SA, et al. The 2016 revision of the World Health Organization classification of lymphoid neoplasms. Blood. 2016;127:2375–90.
3. Hutchings M, Loft A, Hansen M, et al. FDG-PET after two cycles of chemotherapy predicts treatment failure and progression-free survival in Hodgkin lymphoma. Blood. 2006;107:52–9.
4. Safar V, Dupuis J, Itti E, et al. Interim [18F]fluorodeoxyglucose positron emission tomography scan in diffuse large B-cell lymphoma treated with anthracycline-based chemotherapy plus rituximab. J Clin Oncol. 2012;30:184–90.
5. Pregno P, Chiappella A, Bellò M, et al. Interim 18-FDG-PET/CT failed to predict the outcome in diffuse large B-cell lymphoma patients treated at the diagnosis with rituximab-CHOP. Blood. 2012;119:2066–73.
6. Cheson BD, Fisher RI, Barrington SF, Cavalli F, Schwartz LH, Zucca E, Lister TA. Recommendations for initial evaluation, staging, and response assessment of Hodgkin and non-Hodgkin lymphoma: the Lugano classification. J Clin Oncol. 2014;32:3059–67.
7. Fisher RI. The New England Journal of Medicine. No other uses without permission. Copyright © 1993 Massachusetts Medical Society. All rights reserved. N Engl J Med. 1993;29:1230–5.
8. Ziepert M, Hasenclever D, Kuhnt E, Glass B, Schmitz N, Pfreundschuh M, Loeffler M. Standard international prognostic index remains a valid predictor of outcome for patients with aggressive CD20+ B-cell lymphoma in the rituximab era. J Clin Oncol. 2010;28:2373–80.
9. Zhou Z, Sehn LH, Rademaker AW, et al. An enhanced International Prognostic Index (NCCN-IPI) for patients with diffuse large B-cell lymphoma treated in the rituximab era. Blood. 2014;123:837–42.

10. Solal-Céligny P, Roy P, Colombat P, et al. Follicular lymphoma international prognostic index. Blood. 2004;104:1258–65.
11. Hoster E, Dreyling M, Klapper W, et al. A new prognostic index (MIPI) for patients with advanced-stage mantle cell lymphoma. Blood. 2008;111:558–65.
12. Junlén HR, Peterson S, Kimby E, et al. Follicular lymphoma in Sweden: nationwide improved survival in the rituximab era, particularly in elderly women: a Swedish Lymphoma Registry Study. Leukemia. 2015;29:668–76.
13. Harris NL, Jaffe ES, Diebold J, Flandrin G, Muller-Hermelink HK, Vardiman J, Lister TA, Bloomfield CD. World health organization classification of neoplastic diseases of the hematopoietic and lymphoid tissues: report of the clinical advisory committee meeting—Airlie house, Virginia, November 1997. J Clin Oncol. 1999;17:3835–49.
14. Nguyen LN, Ha CS, Hess M, Romaguera JE, Manning JT, Cabanillas F, Cox JD. The outcome of combined-modality treatments for stage I and II primary large B-cell lymphoma of the mediastinum. Int J Radiat Oncol Biol Phys. 2000;47:1281–5.
15. Achten R, Verhoef G, Vanuytsel L, De Wolf-Peeters C. T-cell/Histiocyte–rich large B-cell lymphoma: a distinct Clinicopathologic entity. J Clin Oncol. 2002;20:1269–77.
16. Bhagavathi S, Wilson JD. Primary central nervous system lymphoma. Arch Pathol Lab Med. 2008;132(11):1830–4. https://doi.org/10.1043/1543-2165-132.11.1830.
17. Ferreri AJM, Blay JY, Reni M, et al. Prognostic scoring system for primary CNS lymphomas: the International Extranodal Lymphoma Study Group experience. J Clin Oncol. 2003;21:266–72.
18. Novak U, Basso K, Pasqualucci L, Dalla-Favera R, Bhagat G. Genomic analysis of non-splenic marginal zone lymphomas (MZL) indicates similarities between nodal and extranodal MZL and supports their derivation from memory B-cells. Br J Haematol. 2011;155:362–5.
19. Sagaert X, De Wolf-Peeters C, Noels H, Baens M. The pathogenesis of MALT lymphomas: where do we stand? Leukemia. 2007;21:389–96.

Pathology of Non-Hodgkin Lymphomas

2

Sridhar Epari

Contents

2.1 Introduction

Lymphomas are a heterogenous group of malignancies of lymphoid tissue with diversity in cellular origin, morphology, immunophenotype, cytogenetics, molecular abnormalities, differential treatment response, and prognosis. They are characterized by clonal proliferation of mature and immature lymphoid cells, primarily involve lymphoreticular organs and can also populate bone marrow/blood. Primary presentation with involvement of the bone marrow and/or blood is referred to as leukemias, while those restricted to the lymphatic system are referred to as lymphomas. However, they share common biological features and are not distinct, i.e., overlapping of their presentations can occur which may depend on the stage of the disease, both may have peripheral lymphocytosis and bone marrow involvement. Based on the clinicopathological and biological features, they are classified into two broad categories—Hodgkin and non-Hodgkin lymphoma (Table 2.1). Hodgkin lymphomas are not discussed in this chapter.

S. Epari (✉)
Department of Pathology, Tata Memorial Hospital and ACTREC, Homi Bhabha National Institute, Mumbai, India

15

Table 2.1 Comparison of Hodgkin and non-Hodgkin lymphoma

Features	Hodgkin lymphoma	Non-Hodgkin lymphoma
Histology	The neoplastic cells are in minority and comprise approximately1% of the all cells	The neoplastic cells are the predominant cellular composition
Nodal involvement	Typically localized to a specific group of nodes	Usually disseminated among >1 nodal group
Spread	Contiguous fashion	Non-contiguously
Effect on Waldeyer ring and mesenteric lymph nodes	Usually does not affect	Commonly affects mesenteric nodes May affect Waldeyer ring
Extranodal involvement	Infrequent	Frequent
Stage at diagnosis	Usually early	Usually advanced
Age-group	Bimodal peak; children and young adults more common	Commonly in older and elderly population
Histologic classification in children	Usually one with a favorable prognosis	Usually aggressive

Non-Hodgkin lymphomas (NHLs) are one of the common prevalent cancers. The risk factors for its occurrence include immunological disturbances (autoimmune disorders, chronic inflammatory states, etc.), viral (HIV, EBV, HCV, H. pylori, etc.), environmental (pesticides, herbicides, smoking, etc.) and genetic factors (SCID, Klinefelters, etc.).

2.2   Classification and Diagnosis

Classification of non-Hodgkin lymphoma is continuously evolving which is by itself reflective of continuous emergence of new insights into the biological basis and cell of origin concepts. The 2017 WHO classification is the currently followed system which is essentially in principle with the updated REAL classification, incorporates morphology, immunophenotype, genotype, and cytogenetics for defining an entity [1, 2]. There are more than 60 distinct subtypes of lymphoid cell neoplasms listed in the current WHO classification (Tables 2.2 and 2.3) [1]. Based on the type of lymphocyte or immune cell involved, they are classified either of mature or immature B/T-lymphoid cell types, NK-cell type, and histiocyte/dendritic cell types. These are further subtyped based on the stage of differentiation and biological properties of the neoplastic B-cells, T-cells, or NK-cells, however as NK-cells share certain biological similarities with T-cells are often considered together [3].

The neoplastic cells in most of the B and T-cell neoplasms can be recapitulated to the normal stage of differentiation with few exceptions like hairy cell leukemia, where the corresponding differentiation stage cannot be ascertained (Fig. 2.1) [3]. Based on the differentiation stages, they can be precursor/blastoid lymphoid neoplasms or of mature B and T/NK cell neoplasms (Tables 2.2 and 2.3) The precursor neoplasms can be of leukemic or lymphomatous in presentation but are considered to be spectrum of same biological entity and treated similarly. The B-lymphoblastic is predominantly leukemic but T-lymphoblastic can present either in lymphomatous

Table 2.2 Precursor lymphoid neoplasms listed in the current WHO classification

B-lymphoblastic leukemia/lymphoma, NOS
B-lymphoblastic leukemia/lymphoma with t(9;22)(q34.1;q11.2); BCR-ABL 1
B-lymphoblastic leukemia/lymphoma with t(v; 11 q23.3); KMT2A-rearranged
B-lymphoblastic leukemia/lymphoma with t(12;21)(p13.2;q22.1); ETV6-RUNX1
B-lymphoblastic leukemia/lymphoma with hyperdiploidy
B-lymphoblastic leukemia/lymphoma with hypodiploidy (hypodiploid ALL)
B-lymphoblastic leukemia/lymphoma with t(5;14)(q31.1;q32.1); IGH/IL3
B-lymphoblastic leukemia/lymphoma with t(1;19)(q23;p13.3); TCF3-PBX1
B-lymphoblastic leukemia/lymphoma, BCR-ABL1-like
B-lymphoblastic leukemia/lymphoma with lymphoma iAMP21
T-lymphoblastic leukemia/lymphoma
Early T-cell precursor lymphoblastic leukemia
NK-lymphoblastic leukemia/lymphoma[a]

[a]Listed as provisional entity in the current 2017 WHO classification

or leukemic forms. The mature B-cell NHLs are more prevalent, the T/NK-cell-NHLs are uncommon, while the histiocyte/dendritic cell tumors are rare.

Diagnosis of the non-Hodgkin lymphomas is essentially based on the microscopic examination of the involved tissue/bone marrow/blood, which include the basic evaluation for morphological features, immunophenotypic (immunohistochemistry on tissue, while flow cytometry on fluid samples) characterization, and cytogenetic/molecular characterization, wherever it is indicated.

1. *Morphological features*: Microscopic evaluation for various features forms the cornerstone in evaluation for lymphomas. The features need to be evaluated are patterns of the effacement (diffuse/partial/sinusoidal, etc.), architecture of the disease (diffuse/follicular/nodular), composition of the neoplastic cells (monomorphous/polymorphous), type/size of the neoplastic cells (blastoid/non-blastoid, small, intermediate or large-sized, centroblastic, immunoblastic, plasmablastic, etc.), and other features (mitotic activity, necrosis, angiocentricity, etc.). These features serve as the basis for further characterization.

2. *Immunophenotypic evaluation*: Done for lineage determination and helps in establishing stage of the maturation of the neoplastic cells. It is done by immunohistochemistry (IHC) and/or flow cytometry (FCM)—IHC is normally performed on formalin-fixed and paraffin-embedded tissue and FCM can be evaluated only on fresh unfixed tissue/fluid samples. FCM has the advantage of being faster and better at simultaneously identifying co-expression of multiple markers on the same cell populations. However, certain markers can only be evaluated by IHC. The characterization of lymphomas into B-, T-, or NK-cell types is by immunophenotypic analysis and also for further typing. Typical pan B-cell antigens include PAX5, CD19, CD20, and CD79a and typical pan T-cell antigens include CD2, CD5, and CD7. The precursor or blastic immature lymphomas express one or more of TdT and/or CD34 (T-lymphoblastic lymphoma may also co-express CD1a).

3. *Cytogenetic and Molecular evaluation* can help in cases where the morphologic and immunophenotypic analysis is inconclusive or indeterminate—e.g.,

Table 2.3   2016 WHO classification of mature lymphoid cell neoplasms

Mature B-cell neoplasms
Chronic lymphocytic leukemia/small lymphocytic lymphoma
Monoclonal B-cell lymphocytosis
B-cell prolymphocytic leukemia
Splenic marginal zone lymphoma
Hairy cell leukemia
Splenic B-cell lymphoma/leukemia, unclassifiable
  Splenic diffuse red pulp small B-cell lymphoma
  Hairy cell leukemia-variant
Lymphoplasmacytic lymphoma
  Waldenström macroglobulinemia
Monoclonal gammopathy of undetermined significance (MGUS), IgM
μ heavy-chain disease
γ heavy-chain disease
α heavy-chain disease
Monoclonal gammopathy of undetermined significance (MGUS), IgG/A
Plasma cell myeloma
Solitary plasmacytoma of bone
Extraosseous plasmacytoma
Monoclonal immunoglobulin deposition diseases
Extranodal marginal zone lymphoma of mucosa-associated lymphoid tissue (MALT lymphoma)
Nodal marginal zone lymphoma
  Pediatric nodal marginal zone lymphoma
Follicular lymphoma
  In situ follicular neoplasia
  Duodenal-type follicular lymphoma
Pediatric-type follicular lymphoma
Large B-cell lymphoma with IRF4 rearrangement
Primary cutaneous follicle center lymphoma
Mantle cell lymphoma
  In situ mantle cell neoplasia
Diffuse large B-cell lymphoma (DLBCL), NOS
  Germinal center B-cell type
  Activated B-cell type
T-cell/histiocyte-rich large B-cell lymphoma
Primary DLBCL of the central nervous system (CNS)
Primary cutaneous DLBCL, leg type
EBV+ DLBCL, NOS
EBV+ mucocutaneous ulcer
DLBCL associated with chronic inflammation
Lymphomatoid granulomatosis
Primary mediastinal (thymic) large B-cell lymphoma
Intravascular large B-cell lymphoma
ALK+ large B-cell lymphoma
Plasmablastic lymphoma
Primary effusion lymphoma
HHV8+ DLBCL, NOS
Burkitt lymphoma
Burkitt-like lymphoma with 11q aberration
High-grade B-cell lymphoma, with MYC and BCL2 and/or BCL6 rearrangements
High-grade B-cell lymphoma, NOS
B-cell lymphoma, unclassifiable, with features intermediate between DLBCL and classical Hodgkin lymphoma

Mature T and NK neoplasms
T-cell prolymphocytic leukemia
T-cell large granular lymphocytic leukemia
Chronic lymphoproliferative disorder of NK-cells
Aggressive NK-cell leukemia
Systemic EBV+ T-cell lymphoma of childhood
Hydroa vacciniforme-like lymphoproliferative disorder
Adult T-cell leukemia/lymphoma
Extranodal NK-/T-cell lymphoma, nasal type
Enteropathy-associated T-cell lymphoma
Monomorphic epitheliotropic intestinal T-cell lymphoma
Indolent T-cell lymphoproliferative disorder of the GI tract
Hepatosplenic T-cell lymphoma
Subcutaneous panniculitis-like T-cell lymphoma
Mycosis fungoides
Sézary syndrome
Primary cutaneous CD30+ T-cell lymphoproliferative disorders
  Lymphomatoid papulosis
  Primary cutaneous anaplastic large-cell lymphoma
Primary cutaneous γδ T-cell lymphoma
Primary cutaneous CD8+ aggressive epidermotropic cytotoxic T-cell lymphoma
Primary cutaneous acral CD8+ T-cell lymphoma
Primary cutaneous CD4+ small/medium T-cell lymphoproliferative disorder
Peripheral T-cell lymphoma, NOS
Angioimmunoblastic T-cell lymphoma
Follicular T-cell lymphoma
Nodal peripheral T-cell lymphoma with TFH phenotype
Anaplastic large-cell lymphoma, ALK+
Anaplastic large-cell lymphoma, ALK−
Breast implant–associated anaplastic large-cell lymphoma

Post-transplant lymphoproliferative disorders (PTLD)
Plasmacytic hyperplasia PTLD
Infectious mononucleosis PTLD
Florid follicular hyperplasia PTLD
Polymorphic PTLD
Monomorphic PTLD (B- and T-/NK-cell types)
Classical Hodgkin lymphoma PTLD

a   **b**

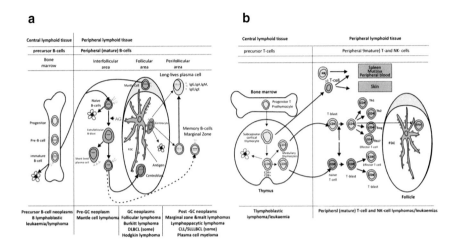

Fig. 2.1 Normal B-cell (**a**) and T-cell (**b**) differentiation and its relationship to their corresponding neoplasm (although the normal cell counterparts are unknown in some instances). The red bars indicate IGH gene rearrangement and the blue bars IG light chain gene rearrangement; the black insertions in red and blue bars indicate somatic hypermutation Recently recognized T-cell subsets include the various types of CD4+ effector T-cells, including T helper 1 (Th1), T helper 2 (Th2), T regulatory (Treg), T helper 17 (Th17), and T follicular helper (TFH) cells. *AG* antigen, *CLL/SLL* chronic lymphocytic leukemia/small lymphocytic lymphoma, *D* surface IgD, *DLBCL* diffuse large 8-cell lymphoma, *FDC* follicular dendritic cell, *M* surface IgM, *MALT* mucosa-associated lymphoid tissue. (Modified from Swerdlow et al., WHO classification of tumors of hematopoietic and lymphoid tissues. Revised fourth ed. 2017)

Table 2.4 List of common lymphomas with associated chromosomal translocations

Lymphoma type	Translocation	Percentage affected	Proto-oncogene
Follicular lymphoma	t(14;18)(q32;q21)	90%	BCL2
	t(2;18)(p11;q21)		
	t(18;22)(q21;q11)		
Mantle cell lymphoma	t(11;14)(q13;q32)	70%	Cyclin D1
Burkitt lymphoma	t(8;14)(q24;q32)	80%	CMYC
	t(2;8)(p11;q24)	15%	
	t(8;22)(q24;q11)	5%	
Anaplastic large-cell lymphoma	t(2;5)(p23;q35)	60% in adults	NPM/ALK
		85% in children	
MALT lymphomas	t(11;18)(q21;q21)	50%	API2/MLT
	t(1;14)(p22;q32)	Rare	BCL10

molecular analyses for the rearrangements of the variable region of the immuno-globulin (IG) or T-cell receptor (TCR) genes (to determine clonal or polyclonal), specific gene rearrangements by FISH (t(14;18)/*IGH-BCL2* in follicular lymphomas, MYC/BCL2/BCL6 for double/triple- hit lymphomas) and mutations on specific genes (*MYD88* in lymphoplasmacytic lymphoma and *BRAFV600E* for hairy cell leukemia) (Table 2.4).

2.2.1 B-Cell Non-Hodgkin Lymphomas

Nearly 80–90% of the all NHLs are of mature B-cell origin, they are a heterogeneous group of neoplasms with more than 30 listed entities in the WHO 2017 classification. They typically express pan B-cell markers with surface membrane immunoglobulin. Most of these can be classified based on the resemblance to the stages of differentiation, thus can be identified by a distinctive immunophenotype. Some of them express markers that are not akin to normal mature B-cells, e.g., cyclin D1 in mantle cell lymphoma, BCL2 in germinal center B-cells in follicular lymphoma. This typical immunophenotype along with the morphological features helps for definite diagnosis of each of the subtype (Table 2.5). The common mature B-cell lymphomas include diffuse large B-cell lymphoma (DLBCL), follicular lymphoma, small lymphocytic lymphoma, mantle cell lymphoma, marginal zone lymphoma, Burkitt lymphoma, and lymphoplasmacytic lymphoma.

Based on the clinical behavior, the B-NHLs broadly can be classified as aggressive (intermediate and high grade) and indolent (low grade), which histologically corresponds to large cell/blastoid and small cell cytomorphologies, respectively (Table 2.6). DLBCL and follicular lymphomas are commonest high-grade and low-grade B-NHLs. With exception of the mantle cell lymphomas, all aggressive B-cell NHLs show large cell or blastoid morphology with easily identifiable mitotic activity and are usually characterized by high MIB-1 labeling index (of at least >40%), while the indolent B-NHLs show small to intermediate-sized lymphoid cells with either diffuse or nodular/follicular architecture. Combining the morphological details (especially cell size and architecture, i.e., diffuse/follicular nature) along with distinctive immunophenotypic findings, different subsets of low grade/indolent B-cell lymphomas can be diagnosis. One such algorithmic immunophenotypic approach is shown in Fig. 2.2.

Whereas for high-grade B-cell NHLs, the current WHO classification lists the entities and also provided a schematic diagnostic algorithm (Table 2.7). All de novo high-grade mature B-cell non-Hodgkin lymphomas with *MYC* and *BCL2* and/or *BCL6* gene rearrangements are classified as double/triple-hit (DH/TH) lymphomas. The diagnosis of DLBCL, NOS should be made only after the exclusion of the DH/THL and the special types of large B-cell lymphomas, which then subtyped further on morphological features (centroblastic, immunoblastic, and anaplastic) and/or cell of-origin (COO) basis (germinal center B-cell [GCB] subtype and activated B-cell [ABC] subtype). The COO subtyping is typically done by differential gene expression; immunohistochemical-based method using Hans algorithm also showed good concordance (Fig. 2.3). Additionally, based on the co-expression of MYC and BCL2 protein on IHC (BCL2 is considered positive if>50% of the tumor cells are positive and MYC is considered positive if >40% of the tumor cell nuclei are positive), are assigned as double expressers (DE), which is seen more commonly in the ABC subtype [1]. However, it is to be noted that MYC protein expression cannot be used to predict the presence of *MYC* gene rearrangement, though the cutoff value of 70% has been recently reported to be reproducible among different centers and of clinical value in identifying patients with a worse prognosis [4, 5]. However, it is

Table. 2.5 Immunophenotypic features of common mature B-cell neoplasms

Neoplasm		slg, clg	CD5	CD10	CD23	CD43	CD103	BCL6	MUM1	Cyclin D1	Annexin A1
CLL/SLL	Indolent/Low grade	+, -/+	+	-	+	+	-	-	+ (PCs)	-	-
LPL		+/-, +	-[c]	-	-	-/+	-	-	+[a]	-	-
SMZL		+, -/+	-	-	-	-	-	-	-	-	-
HCL		+, -	-	-	-	-	+	-	-	+/-	+
PCM[f]		-, +	-	-/+	-	-/+	-	-	+[a]	-/+	-
MALT lymphoma	Indolent/Low grade	+, +/-	-[c]	-	-	-/+	-	-	+[a]	-	-
FL[f]		+, -	-[c]	+/-	-/+	-	-	+	-/+[b]	-	-
MCL[f]	Intermediate grade	+, -	+	-	-	+	-	-	-	+	-
DLBCL	Aggressive/High	+/-, -/+	-[c]	-/+[d]	n/a	-/+	n/a	+/-[d]	+/-[e]	-	-
BL	grade	+, -	-	+	-	-/+	n/a	+	-/+	-	-

>90% (+), >50% (+/-), <50% (-/+), or <10% (-)

BL Burkitt lymphoma, clg cytoplasmic immunoglobulin, CLL/SLL chronic lymphocytic leukemia/ small lymphocytic lymphoma, DLBCL diffuse large B-cell lymphoma, FL follicular lymphoma, HICL hairy cell leukemia, LPL lymphoplasmacytic lymphoma, MALT mucosa-associated lymphoid tissue, MCL mantle cell lymphoma, n/a not applicable, PC proliferation center, PCM plasma cell myeloma, slg surface immunoglobulin, SMZL splenic marginal zone lymphoma

[a] The plasma cell components of LPL and MALT lymphoma are MUM+
[b] Some grade 3A and 3B FLs are MUM+
[c] Some DLBCLs are CD5+. Other B-cell neoplasms can sometimes be CD5+, including LPL, MALT, and FL
[d] DLBCLs of germinal center-B-ceU type express CD10 and BCL6
[e] DLBCLs of activated B-cell type are typically MUM+
[f] Some subtypes have aggressive behavior/high-grade morphology

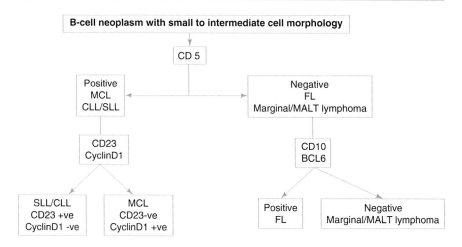

Fig. 2.2 A practical algorithmic approach for small B-cell neoplasms. *CLL* Chronic lymphocytic leukemia, *FL* Follicular lymphoma, *MCL* Mantle cell lymphoma, *SLL* Small lymphocytic lymphoma

Table 2.6 List of common aggressive and indolent lymphomas

Aggressive lymphomas	Indolent lymphomas
B-cell types	B-cell types
• Burkitt lymphoma and Burkitt-like lymphoma	• Small lymphocytic lymphoma/chronic lymphocytic leukemia (SLL/CLL).
• Diffuse large B-cell lymphoma	• Follicular lymphoma
• Primary mediastinal large B-cell lymphomas	• Hairy cell leukemia
• AIDS-associated lymphomas and post-transplant lymphoproliferative disorders	• Lymphoplasmacytic lymphoma/ Waldenstrom macroglobulinemia
• All other subtypes of large B-cell non-Hodgkin lymphomas	• Marginal zone—Nodal
• Lymphoblastic lymphoma	• Splenic marginal zone lymphoma
• Mantle cell lymphoma (sometimes behaves indolently)	T-cell types
T-cell types	• Mycosis fungoides
• Peripheral T-cell lymphoma	• T-CLL
• Lymphoblastic lymphoma	• T-cell large granular leukemia
• Anaplastic large-cell lymphoma	

routine practice to evaluate for DH/THL in cases of B-cell lymphomas of blastoid morphology with negativity for cyclin D1 and precursor markers (Tdt and CD34) and in cases with morphological features intermediate between Burkitt lymphoma and DLBCL. In these cases without *MYC* translocation, evaluation (FISH) for chromosome 11q may be advised to rule out the possibility of Burkitt-like lymphoma with 11q aberrations (Fig. 2.4).

Table 2.7 2017 WHO classification (revised fourth edition) listed mature large B-cell non-Hodgkin lymphomas

Diffuse large B-cell lymphoma, NOS
    Morphological variants
        Centroblastic
        Lmmunoblastic
        Anaplastic
        Other rare variants
    Molecular subtypes
        Germinal center B-cell subtype
        Activated B-cell subtype
Other lymphomas of large B-cells
    T-cell/histiocyte-rich large B-cell lymphoma
    Primary diffuse large B-cell lymphoma of the CNS
    Primary cutaneous diffuse large B-cell lymphoma, leg type
    EBV-positive diffuse large B-cell lymphoma, NOS
    Diffuse large B-cell lymphoma associated with chronic inflammation
    Lymphomatoid granulomatosis
    Large B-cell lymphoma with IRF4 rearrangement
    Primary mediastinal (thymic) large B-cell lymphoma
    Intravascular large B-cell lymphoma
    ALK-positive large B-cell lymphoma
    Plasmablastic lymphoma
    HHVB-positive diffuse large B-cell lymphoma
    Primary effusion lymphoma
High-grade B-cell lymphoma
    High-grade B-cell lymphoma with MYC and BCL2 and/or BCL6 rearrangements
    High-grade B-cell lymphoma, NOS
B-cell lymphoma, unclassifiable
    B-cell lymphoma, unclassifiable, with features intermediate between diffuse large B-cell lymphoma and classic Hodgkin lymphoma

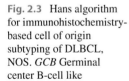 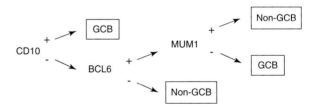

Fig. 2.3 Hans algorithm for immunohistochemistry-based cell of origin subtyping of DLBCL, NOS. *GCB* Germinal center B-cell like

2.2.2 T-Cell Non-Hodgkin Lymphomas

Relatively uncommon and account for approximately 10–15% of all NHL, of which cutaneous types are the commonest [6]. Like the B-cell counterparts they can present predominantly as cutaneous, other extranodal, nodal, and/or leukemias (Fig. 2.5). Tumors of mature T-cells, i.e., post-thymic or peripheral are referred to collectively as peripheral T-cell lymphomas (PTCLs) and while the tumors of precursor T-cell are lymphoblastic lymphomas. The WHO classification lists over 25 definite or

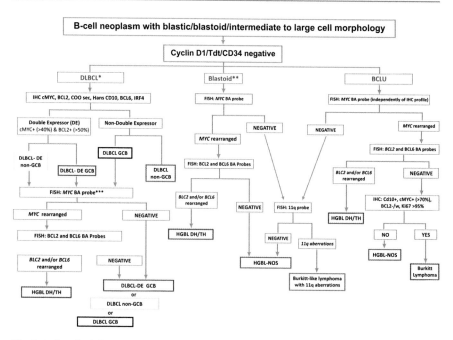

Fig. 2.4 Practical diagnostic algorithmic approach to mature aggressive B-cell lymphoma. This does not for the specific DLBCL entities (i.e., primary mediastinal B-cell lymphoma [PMBCL]), intravascular DLBCL, EBV+ DLBCL, T-cell rich histiocyte-rich B-cell lymphoma (TCRHRBCL), etc. (*) and to blastoid lymphomas excluding lymphoblastic lymphomas and mantle cell lymphomas (**). *BCLU* B-cell lymphoma-unclassifiable, *BL* Burkitt lymphoma, *DH* double hit, *DLBCL* Diffuse large B-cell lymphoma, *GCB* germinal center B-cell, *HGBL* high-grade B-cell lymphoma (Modified from Di Napoli et al. 2019)

provisional entities under the heading of mature T- and NK-cell neoplasms (Table 2.3). Most PTCLs carry a poorer prognosis than the most B-cell counterparts [6, 7]. Except for anaplastic lymphoma kinase (ALK)-positive anaplastic large-cell lymphoma (ALCL), outcomes for most other subtypes of mature T-cell lymphomas are poor.

Mature T-cell lymphomas generally express one or more T-cell markers, and tend to display a T helper (CD4-positive) or cytotoxic (CD8-positive) immunophenotype and may show loss of markers expressed by most normal T-cells (e.g., CD5, CD7). However, a subset of them may express markers not commonly detected in normal T-cells, such as ALK. NK-cell lymphomas lack surface CD3 (expressing only cytoplasmic CD3) and CD5 but express some pan T-cell antigens (such as CD2 and CD7) as well as CD16 and/or CD56. Diagnosis of T-cell lymphomas is usually confirmed by application of IHC/FCM-based antibody panels and if required with further genetic studies. With the expression of the antibodies and morphological features, diagnosis of T-cell lymphomas can be achieved by using a simplistic algorithm (as shown in Fig. 2.6). However, further detailed descriptions and diagnostic criteria is beyond the scope of this chapter.

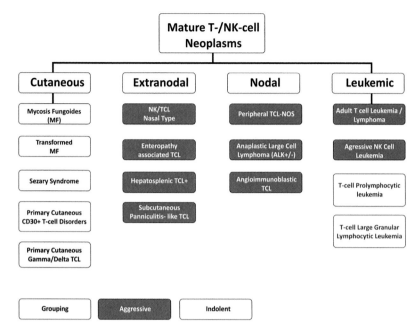

Fig. 2.5 Mature T/NK cell neoplasms: presentation-based entities (Modified from Rodriguez J et al. 2009)

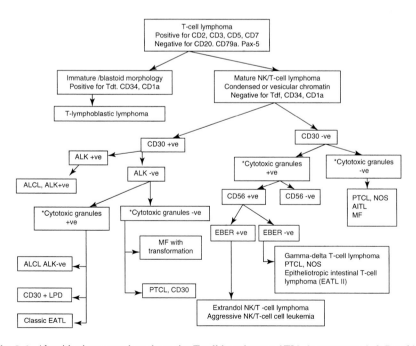

Fig. 2.6 Algorithmic approach to the major T-cell lymphomas. *TIA-1; granzyme A & Perofrin. *ALCL* Anaplastic large-cell lymphoma, *EATL* Enteropathy-associated T-cell lymphoma, *LPD* Lymphoproliferative disorder, *PTCL* Peripheral T-cell lymphoma

References

1. Swerdlow SH, Campo E, Harris NL, Jaffe ES, Pileri SA, Stein H, Thiele J, editors. WHO classification of tumours of haematopoietic and lymphoid tissues. Revised 4th ed. Lyon: IARC; 2017.
2. Harris NL, Jaffe ES, Stein H, et al. A revised European–American classification of lymphoid neoplasms: a proposal from the International Lymphoma Study Group. Blood. 1994;84:1361–92.
3. The non-Hodgkin's lymphoma classification project: a clinical evaluation of the International Lymphoma Study Group classification of non-Hodgkin's lymphoma. Blood. 1997;89(11):3909–3918.
4. Ambrosio MR, Lazzi S, Lo Bello G, et al. MYC protein expression scoring and its impact on the prognosis of aggressive B-cell lymphoma patients. Haematologica. 2019;104(1):e25–8.
5. Di Napoli A, Remotti D, Agostinelli C, Ambrosio MR, Ascani S, Carbone A, Facchetti F, Lazzi S, Leoncini L, Lucioni M, Novero D, Pileri S, Ponzoni M, Sabattini E, Tripodo C, Zamò A, Paulli M, Ruco L. Correction to: a practical algorithmic approach to mature aggressive B cell lymphoma diagnosis in the double/triple hit era: selecting cases, matching clinical benefit. Virchows Arch. 2019;475(6):799.
6. Vose J, Armitage J, Weisenburger D, International T-Cell Lymphoma Project. International peripheral T-cell and natural killer/T-cell lymphoma study: pathology findings and clinical outcomes. J Clin Oncol. 2008;26(25):4124–30.
7. Rodríguez J, Gutiérrez A, Martínez-Delgado B, Perez-Manga G. Current and future aggressive peripheral T-cell lymphoma treatment paradigms, biological features and therapeutic molecular targets. Crit Rev Oncol Hematol. 2009;71(3):181–98.

Management of Non-Hodgkin's Lymphoma

3

Vasu Babu Goli and Manju Sengar

Contents

Management of NHL is guided by the histological subtype, extent or stage of the disease, age, performance status, organ function of the host, and in some cases on the underlying etiology (e.g., HCV-related marginal zone lymphoma, H. pylori related gastric marginal zone lymphoma). The following sections will highlight the management of NHL based on the above-mentioned factors.

V. Babu Goli · M. Sengar (✉)
Department of Medical Oncology, Tata Memorial Hospital, Homi Bhabha National Institute, Mumbai, India

3.1   Follicular Lymphoma (FL)

The therapeutic decision in FL is based on the grade (grade1-3a versus 3b), stage, disease burden, presence of transformation to high-grade B-NHL. The grade 3b disease behaves like and diffuse large B-cell NHL and therefore managed on the same principles (refer to Sect. 3.5).

(a) **Early-stage Follicular Lymphoma:** Stage I/II follicular lymphomas constitute less than 10% of patients [1]. Radiation therapy (24 Gy) is the treatment of choice for early-stage low grade (grade1-3a) follicular lymphoma, where all involved sites can be encompassed in the radiation field, with a 10-year freedom from treatment failure ranging from 41 to 49% [1, 2] and median survival of 19 years [1]. A baseline PET/CT is helpful in early-stage disease patients who are being planned for radiation to rule out disseminated disease. If the disease involves multiple nodal stations that cannot be safely treated with radiation, watchful waiting or single-agent rituximab are other options.

(b) **Advanced-Stage Disease**
   • **Asymptomatic Disease:** Patients with advanced-stage FL with low tumor burden do not require immediate treatment unless they are symptomatic. Watchful waiting remains the standard of care for asymptomatic patients [3–5].
   • **Symptomatic Disease:** Patients with high tumor burden as per BLNI [3], GELF criteria [6], and symptomatic patients are treated with chemoimmunotherapy. Bendamustine and Rituximab (BR) is the preferred first-line treatment in these patients due to its better efficacy and safety profile as compared to R-CHOP [7, 8]. After a median follow-up of 10 years, BR was associated with better overall survival (71% vs 66% p-0.69), improved median time to next treatment (TTNT) with 34% of patients requiring salvage treatment due to progression compared with 54% in R-CHOP arm. Use of maintenance rituximab has shown improved 10-year progression free-survival PFS (51% vs 35%), time to treatment failure (10.5 years vs 4.1 years) without an effect on overall survival in patients treated with induction therapy (R-CHOP [rituximab, cyclophosphamide, doxorubicin, vincristine, prednisolone], R-FCM [rituximab, fludarabine, cyclophosphamide, mitoxantrone], RCVP [rituximab, cyclophosphamide, vincristine, prednisolone]). However, there was higher incidence of Grade 3/4 adverse events with maintenance treatment and there is no clear evidence of efficacy in patients who receive BR as induction [7, 8].

(c) **Relapsed Follicular Lymphoma:** Patients with the early progression of disease (POD), i.e., defined as progression within the first 2 years, have inferior overall survival (5 year OS-50%) compared with patients without early POD (5 year OS-90%) [9]. Patients with relapsed FL should undergo biopsy from the most FDG-avid site to rule out transformation to high-grade lymphoma. Multiple active agents (R-CHOP, R-Lenalidomide, R-CVP, and other novel agents) are available for relapsed FL and the treatment should be tailored based on the prior therapy, progression-free interval, goals of therapy, and risk of adverse events.

3.2 Marginal Zone Lymphomas

(a) **Nodal Marginal Zone Lymphoma:** Asymptomatic/low burden NMZL is observed with a watch and wait strategy. Treatment should be considered in case of B symptoms, cytopenias due to marrow infiltration by lymphoma, rapid enlargement of nodes, bulky disease, and compromise of vital organ function. In patients with NMZL with concomitant HCV infection, antiviral therapy is indicated and it can induce durable remissions [10]. There are no large studies to address the standard of care, but the limited evidence suggests the use of BR or R-Chemotherapy (CHOP, CVP, or fludarabine) can be used in patients with symptomatic and advanced stage disease [11].

(b) **Splenic Marginal Zone Lymphoma:** Active surveillance is indicated for asymptomatic patients. Patients with underlying HCV infection can be treated with antiviral therapy [10]. Rituximab is preferred over splenectomy for symptomatic patients (progressive/symptomatic splenomegaly and/or cytopenias) [12]. Rituximab monotherapy produces response rates of 80%, CR rate of 40%, and 10-year PFS of 60%. For patients with B symptoms (fever, weight loss >10% over 6 months, and night sweats) and significant abdominal lymphadenopathy, chemoimmunotherapy is indicated [13].

(c) **Extranodal Marginal Zone Lymphoma (MALT lymphoma):** Gastric marginal zone lymphoma (Gastric MZL) should be treated initially with Helicobacter pylori (H. pylori) eradication therapy irrespective of stage. Choice of antimicrobial therapy should be offered based on local antibiotic resistance patterns. The outline for the management of Gastric MZL is shown in Fig. 3.1.

The indications for treatment with systemic therapy include overt progression on anti-microbial therapy, deep invasion, nodal involvement, and t (11;18).

3.3 Mantle Cell Lymphoma

A subset of patients with mantle cell lymphoma can be observed with "wait and watch" strategy. These include asymptomatic patients with low tumor burden, non-bulky disease, low Ki-67, and non-blastoid morphology. In these patients, the median overall survival was significantly longer in the observation group compared with the early treatment group (72 vs 52 months $p = 0.041$) [14]. For young physically fit transplant eligible patients who do not fall in the indolent disease subgroup, rituximab and high-dose cytarabine based therapy should be considered for remission induction

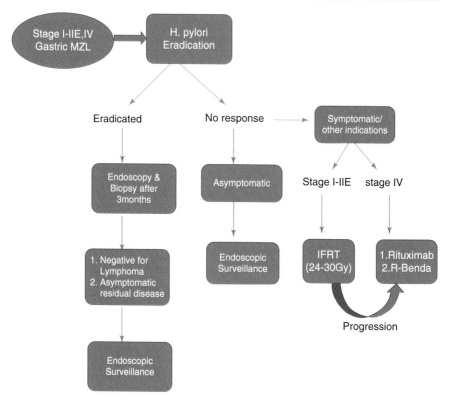

Fig. 3.1 Gastric MALTOMA

followed by autologous stem cell transplantation (ASCT) and rituximab maintenance [15]. In transplant-ineligible patients, Bendamustine-Rituximab (BR) [7] or VR-CAP [16] or RCHOP [8] followed by R maintenance are acceptable treatment options.

3.4 Burkitt Lymphoma

In view of the short doubling time, the treatment requires short-intensive, multi-agent chemotherapy with non-cross resistant drugs. The treatment options include multi-agent high-dose methotrexate-based chemotherapy regimen (CODOX-M/IVAC [cyclophosphamide, vincristine, doxorubicin, high-dose methotrexate/ifosfamide, vincristine, adriamycin, cytarabine] [17], GMALL-B-NHL, etc.) or dose-adjusted-REPOCH-R (etoposide, prednisolone, vincristine, prednisolone, rituximab). For patients with high-risk Burkitt lymphoma without CNS involvement at baseline dose-adjusted R-EPOCH (etoposide, prednisolone, vincristine, prednisolone, rituximab) with intrathecal methotrexate has shown 4-year EFS and

OS of 84.5% and 87%, respectively [18]. Due to inferior event-free survival for patients with CSF involvement and bone marrow involvement with EPOCH-R, GMALL-B-ALL/NHL2002 [19] or CODOX-M/IVAC may be preferable.

3.5   Diffuse Large B-Cell Lymphoma (DLBCL)

Several attempts have been made to improve outcomes of DLBCL with addition of another drug on the R-CHOP backbone, however, none of the regimens has shown better efficacy than R-CHOP.

(a) **Limited stage DLBCL:** Limited stage (stage I/II) DLBCL with favorable prognosis (non-bulky <7.5 cm, normal LDH) can be treated with 4 cycles of R-CHOP (rituximab, cyclophosphamide, doxorubicin, vincristine, predniso-lone) followed by ISRT (RT 30 Gy) for the disease sites where radiation is unlikely to result in significant long-term toxicity [20]. For disease involving mediastinum or breast with the potential of long-term radiation toxicity, 6 cycles of R-CHOP are preferred.

(b) **Advanced-stage DLBCL:** Advanced-stage DLBCL is treated with 6 cycles of R-CHOP [21, 22]. Patients with initial bulky disease (>7.5 cm) and extranodal disease can be consolidated with ISRT after completion of chemoimmunother-apy. However, there is conflicting evidence for consolidative radiation in patients who achieve complete metabolic response with R-CHOP. There is no standard approach for double-hit lymphoma. The retrospective data suggest better outcomes with DA-EPOCH-R [23].

(c) **CNS prophylaxis in DLBCL:** The optimal way to deliver CNS prophylaxis is not clear. Patients with a high risk of CNS relapse (High CNS IPI 4–6, 3 or more extranodal sites (irrespective of CNS IPI) along with high LDH, renal/adrenal or intravascular involvement, breast involvement) with adequate organ function and creatinine clearance of more than 50 mL/min should receive 2–3 cycles of high-dose methotrexate (HD-MTX) 3 g/m^2 infused over 3 h inter-calating with R-CHOP. The addition of HD-MTX was associated with lower CNS relapse in these high-risk patients [24]. Patients unfit for HD-MTX should receive intrathecal methotrexate although there is a lack of evidence to support this approach.

(d) **Relapsed/Refractory DLBCL:** Salvage chemotherapy followed by high-dose therapy and ASCT is the standard of care for relapsed DLBCL. Salvage therapy for relapsed DLBCL includes R-DHAP (rituximab, dexamethasone, high-dose cytarabine, cisplatin), R-GDP (rituximab, gemcitabine, dexamethasone, cispla-tin), R-ICE (rituximab, ifosfamide, carboplatin, etoposide). There is no clear evidence regarding the superiority of one regimen over others [25]. For patients who are not fit for ASCT, options include polatuzumab with BR [26], selinexor [27], or palliative treatment.

3.6 Primary Mediastinal B-Cell Lymphoma (PMBCL)

Most patients with primary mediastinal B-cell lymphoma present with disease localized to the supra-diaphragmatic area. DA-EPOCH-R (etoposide, prednisolone, vincristine, prednisolone, rituximab) is the recommended therapy in view of the excellent EFS and OS of 93% and 97%, respectively [28]. This regimen allows the omission of radiation in patients who achieve a complete metabolic response. Persistent uptake on PET/CT (DS-4) after chemotherapy can be observed with repeat PET/CT after 6–8 weeks as it does not always represent viable disease and shows resolution over time. Approximately 10–30% of patients with PBMCL relapse within the first year of treatment completion. These patients can be managed with salvage therapy followed by ASCT [29]. Pembrolizumab is associated with high response rates, durable activity in relapsed/refractory PMBCL who have failed two lines of therapy [30].

3.7 HIV Associated Diffuse Large B-Cell Lymphomas

The current treatment strategy for this population of patients includes R-CHOP [31], dose-adjusted EPOCH-R (etoposide, prednisolone, vincristine, prednisolone, rituximab) [32] or short course-EPOCH-RR. The advantage of SC-RR-EPOCH includes the need for only three courses of chemotherapy in most patients as 78.7% achieve a complete response after two cycles [33]. All these patients require CNS prophylaxis given the high-risk of CNS relapses. Management of plasmablastic lymphoma is less well defined and outcomes are poor. As they are CD-20 negative treatment options include CHOP or DA-EPOCH [34].

3.8 Primary CNS-Lymphoma (PCNSL)

All patients with primary CNS-lymphoma should undergo complete work up to rule out systemic involvement (PET/CT and bone marrow examination) as well as ocular involvement (slit-lamp examination) and underlying HIV infection. In immunocompetent and fit patients, HD-MTX based combination chemotherapy is used for induction. It produces CR rates of 30–60% treated alone [35, 36] or in combination with other chemotherapeutic agents. The addition of rituximab and cytarabine has shown improvement in outcomes [37]. Consolidation strategies include high-dose chemotherapy, ASCT [38, 39] or multi-agent intensive chemotherapy [40] in patients who are young and in good general condition. The role of whole-brain radiation is limited to patients who do not achieve a complete response after induction or patients who are not fit for intensive induction. Patients ineligible for HD-MTX due to poor performance status, inadequate organ function, or age are treated with rituximab with temozolomide or whole-brain radiotherapy.

3.9   T-Cell Lymphomas

(a) **PTCL NOS, ALK-positive and ALK-negative Anaplastic large-cell lymphoma**: CHOP (cyclophosphamide, doxorubicin, vincristine, prednisolone) or CHOEP (etoposide added to CHOP) are the most commonly used regimen for this subgroup of patients. The addition of etoposide to CHOP improved PFS in patients with age less <60 years and normal LDH. International T lymphoma study group and smaller retrospective studies reported OS rates between 30 and 45% and PFS rates of 20–30% in these subtypes [41]. The 5-year PFS and overall survival for ALK-positive ALCL with CHOP range from 72–82% to 70–90%, respectively. The 5-year PFS and overall survival for ALK-negative ALCL with CHOP range from 36–48% to 40–58%, respectively [42–44]. Recently, the FDA has approved CHP with brentuximab vedotin in CD30 positive PTCL based on the ECHELON-2 trial. In ECHELON 2, CHP-BV (cyclophosphamide, doxorubicin, prednisolone, brentuximab vedotin) produced significantly superior PFS over CHOP [45]. In patients with advanced disease, high failure rates are observed even after the achievement of complete response. Consolidation with ASCT in these patients may improve PFS and OS [46–48]. Hence young fit patients may be counseled for consolidation with ASCT in CR1.

(b) **NK-T-cell lymphoma:**
- **Early-stage localized nasal/extra-nasal NK-T-cell lymphoma:** (stage I/II): Non-MDR dependent drugs together with radiotherapy have produced superior ORR, PFS, and OS in this subtype of T-cell NHL. Various non-MDR dependent regimens include 2/3DeVIC (dexamethasone, etoposide, ifosfamide, and carboplatin) [49], VIPD (etoposide, ifosfamide, cisplatin, and dexamethasone) [50], LVP regimen (l-asparaginase, vincristine, and prednisolone) [51], and GELOX (gemcitabine, l-asparaginase, and oxaliplatin) [52]. Radiotherapy can be used concurrently or as sandwich therapy with chemotherapy. Both approaches give comparable results. Radiotherapy is better tolerated when given in patients who achieve CR and have completed chemotherapy, hence many clinicians tend to use it sequentially after chemotherapy. For patients with comorbidities and unfit patients who cannot tolerate chemotherapy, RT alone can be considered.
- **Advanced-stage NK-T-cell Lymphoma:** Combination chemotherapy remained mainstay of treatment for advanced-stage disease. L-asparaginase based combination regimens are recommended. SMILE (dexamethasone, methotrexate, ifosfamide, L-asparaginase, etoposide) regimen is most commonly used with ORR, CR, and 5- year OS of 80%, 64%, and 52%, respectively [53]. The role of transplantation in consolidation after frontline therapy is controversial.

3.10 Summary

Treatment of NHL has seen significant evolution over the years. The key to delivering optimal therapy remains accurate diagnosis, proper staging, careful assessment of host and maintaining the desired dose intensity of therapy.

References

1. Friedberg J, Huang J, Dillon H, Farber C, Feliciano S, Hainsworth J, et al. Initial therapeutic strategy in follicular lymphoma (FL): an analysis from the National LymphoCare Study (NLCS). J Clin Oncol. 2006;24:428S.
2. Mac Manus MP, Hoppe RT. Is radiotherapy curative for stage I and II low-grade follicular lymphoma? Results of a long-term follow-up study of patients treated at Stanford University. J Clin Oncol. 14(4):1282–90.
3. Ardeshna KM, Smith P, Norton A, Hancock BW, Hoskin PJ, MacLennan KA, et al. Long-term effect of a watch and wait policy versus immediate systemic treatment for asymptomatic advanced-stage non-Hodgkin lymphoma: a randomised controlled trial. Lancet. 2003;362(9383):516–22.
4. Solal-Céligny P, Bellei M, Marcheselli L, Pesce EA, Pileri S, McLaughlin P, et al. Watchful waiting in low-tumor burden follicular lymphoma in the rituximab era: results of an F2-study database. J Clin Oncol. 2012;30(31):3848–53.
5. Ardeshna KM, Qian W, Smith P, Braganca N, Lowry L, Patrick P, et al. Rituximab versus a watch-and-wait approach in patients with advanced-stage, asymptomatic, non-bulky follicular lymphoma: an open-label randomised phase 3 trial. Lancet Oncol. 2014;15(4):424–35.
6. Brice P, Bastion Y, Lepage E, Brousse N, Haïoun C, Moreau P, et al. Comparison in low-tumor-burden follicular lymphomas between an initial no-treatment policy, prednimustine, or interferon alfa: a randomized study from the Groupe d'Etude des Lymphomes Folliculaires. Groupe d'Etude des Lymphomes de l'Adulte. J Clin Oncol. 1997;15(3):1110–7.
7. Salles G, Seymour JF, Offner F, López-Guillermo A, Belada D, Xerri L, et al. Rituximab maintenance for 2 years in patients with high tumour burden follicular lymphoma responding to rituximab plus chemotherapy (PRIMA): a phase 3, randomised controlled trial. Lancet. 2011;377(9759):42–51.
8. Bachy E, Seymour JF, Feugier P, Offner F, López-Guillermo A, Belada D, et al. Sustained progression-free survival benefit of rituximab maintenance in patients with follicular lymphoma: long-term results of the PRIMA study. JCO. 2019;37(31):2815–24.
9. Casulo C, Byrtek M, Dawson KL, Zhou X, Farber CM, Flowers CR, et al. Early relapse of follicular lymphoma after rituximab plus cyclophosphamide, doxorubicin, vincristine, and prednisone defines patients at high risk for death: an analysis from the National LymphoCare Study. JCO. 2015;33(23):2516–22.
10. Arcaini L, Vallisa D, Rattotti S, Ferretti VV, Ferreri AJM, Bernuzzi P, et al. Antiviral treatment in patients with indolent B-cell lymphomas associated with HCV infection: a study of the Fondazione Italiana Linfomi. Ann Oncol. 2014;25(7):1404–10.
11. Brown JR, Friedberg JW, Feng Y, Scofield S, Phillips K, Dal Cin P, et al. A phase 2 study of concurrent fludarabine and rituximab for the treatment of marginal zone lymphomas. Br J Haematol. 2009;145(6):741–8.
12. Kalpadakis C, Pangalis GA, Dimopoulou MN, Vassilakopoulos TP, Kyrtsonis M-C, Korkolopoulou P, et al. Rituximab monotherapy is highly effective in splenic marginal zone lymphoma. Hematol Oncol. 2007;25(3):127–31.
13. Rummel M, Kaiser U, Balser C, Stauch M, Brugger W, Welslau M, et al. Bendamustine plus rituximab versus fludarabine plus rituximab for patients with relapsed indolent and mantle-cell

lymphomas: a multicentre, randomised, open-label, non-inferiority phase 3 trial. Lancet Oncol. 2016;17(1):57–66.

14. Abrisqueta P, Scott DW, Slack GW, Steidl C, Mottok A, Gascoyne RD, et al. Observation as the initial management strategy in patients with mantle cell lymphoma. Ann Oncol. 2017;28(10):2489–95.

15. Hermine O, Hoster E, Walewski J, Bosly A, Stilgenbauer S, Thieblemont C, et al. Addition of high-dose cytarabine to immunochemotherapy before autologous stem-cell transplantation in patients aged 65 years or younger with mantle cell lymphoma (MCL Younger): a randomised, open-label, phase 3 trial of the European Mantle Cell Lymphoma Network. Lancet. 2016;388(10044):565–75.

16. Robak T, Jin J, Pylypenko H, Verhoef G, Siritanaratkul N, Drach J, et al. Frontline bortezomib, rituximab, cyclophosphamide, doxorubicin, and prednisone (VR-CAP) versus rituximab, cyclophosphamide, doxorubicin, vincristine, and prednisone (R-CHOP) in transplantation-ineligible patients with newly diagnosed mantle cell lymphoma: final overall survival results of a randomised, open-label, phase 3 study. Lancet Oncol. 2018;19(11):1449–58.

17. Mead GM, Sydes MR, Walewski J, Grigg A, Hatton CS, Pescosta N, et al. An international evaluation of CODOX-M and CODOX-M alternating with IVAC in adult Burkitt's lymphoma: results of United Kingdom Lymphoma Group LY06 study. Ann Oncol. 2002;13(8):1264–74.

18. Roschewski M, Dunleavy K, Abramson JS, Powell BL, Link BK, Patel P, et al. Multicenter study of risk-adapted therapy with dose-adjusted epoch-R in adults with untreated Burkitt lymphoma. J Clin Oncol [Internet]. 2020 [cited 2020 Nov 29]. https://ascopubs.org/doi/pdf/10.1200/JCO.20.00303

19. Hoelzer D, Walewski J, Döhner H, Viardot A, Hiddemann W, Spiekermann K, et al. Improved outcome of adult Burkitt lymphoma/leukemia with rituximab and chemotherapy: report of a large prospective multicenter trial. Blood. 2014;124(26):3870–9.

20. Lamy T, Damaj G, Soubeyran P, Gyan E, Cartron G, Bouabdallah K, et al. R-CHOP 14 with or without radiotherapy in nonbulky limited-stage diffuse large B-cell lymphoma. Blood. 2018;131(2):174–81.

21. Pfreundschuh M, Kuhnt E, Trümper L, Osterborg A, Trneny M, Shepherd L, et al. CHOP-like chemotherapy with or without rituximab in young patients with good-prognosis diffuse large-B-cell lymphoma: 6-year results of an open-label randomised study of the MabThera International Trial (MInT) Group. Lancet Oncol. 2011;12(11):1013–22.

22. Coiffier B, Thieblemont C, Van Den Neste E, Lepeu G, Plantier I, Castaigne S, et al. Long-term outcome of patients in the LNH-98.5 trial, the first randomized study comparing rituximab-CHOP to standard CHOP chemotherapy in DLBCL patients: a study by the Groupe d'Etudes des Lymphomes de l'Adulte. Blood. 2010;116(12):2040–5.

23. Oki Y, Noorani M, Lin P, Davis RE, Neelapu SS, Ma L, et al. Double hit lymphoma: the MD Anderson Cancer Center clinical experience. Br J Haematol. 2014;166(6):891–901.

24. Cheah CY, Herbert KE, O'Rourke K, Kennedy GA, George A, Fedele PL, et al. A multicentre retrospective comparison of central nervous system prophylaxis strategies among patients with high-risk diffuse large B-cell lymphoma. Br J Cancer. 2014;111(6):1072–9.

25. Gisselbrecht C, Glass B, Mounier N, Singh Gill D, Linch DC, Trneny M, et al. Salvage regimens with autologous transplantation for relapsed large B-cell lymphoma in the rituximab era. J Clin Oncol. 2010;28(27):4184–90.

26. Sehn LH, Herrera AF, Flowers CR, Kamdar MK, McMillan A, Hertzberg M, et al. Polatuzumab vedotin in relapsed or refractory diffuse large B-cell lymphoma. J Clin Oncol. 2020;38(2):155–65.

27. Kalakonda N, Maerevoet M, Cavallo F, Follows G, Goy A, Vermaat JSP, et al. Selinexor in patients with relapsed or refractory diffuse large B-cell lymphoma (SADAL): a single-arm, multinational, multicentre, open-label, phase 2 trial. Lancet Haematol. 2020;7(7):e511–22.

28. Dunleavy K, Pittaluga S, Maeda LS, Advani R, Chen CC, Hessler J, et al. Dose-adjusted EPOCH-rituximab therapy in primary mediastinal B-cell lymphoma. N Engl J Med. 2013;368(15):1408–16.

29. Aoki T, Shimada K, Suzuki R, Izutsu K, Tomita A, Maeda Y, et al. High-dose chemotherapy followed by autologous stem cell transplantation for relapsed/refractory primary mediastinal large B-cell lymphoma. Blood Cancer J. 2015;5(12):e372.
30. Armand P, Rodig S, Melnichenko V, Thieblemont C, Bouabdallah K, Tumyan G, et al. Pembrolizumab in relapsed or refractory primary mediastinal large B-cell lymphoma. JCO. 2019;37(34):3291–9.
31. Kaplan LD, Lee JY, Ambinder RF, Sparano JA, Cesarman E, Chadburn A, et al. Rituximab does not improve clinical outcome in a randomized phase 3 trial of CHOP with or without rituximab in patients with HIV-associated non-Hodgkin lymphoma: AIDS-malignancies consortium trial 010. Blood. 2005;106(5):1538–43.
32. Little RF, Pittaluga S, Grant N, Steinberg SM, Kavlick MF, Mitsuya H, et al. Highly effective treatment of acquired immunodeficiency syndrome-related lymphoma with dose-adjusted EPOCH: impact of antiretroviral therapy suspension and tumor biology. Blood. 2003;101(12):4653–9.
33. Dunleavy K, Little RF, Pittaluga S, Grant N, Wayne AS, Carrasquillo JA, et al. The role of tumor histogenesis, FDG-PET, and short-course EPOCH with dose-dense rituximab (SC-EPOCH-RR) in HIV-associated diffuse large B-cell lymphoma. Blood. 2010;115(15):3017–24.
34. Castillo JJ, Bibas M, Miranda RN. The biology and treatment of plasmablastic lymphoma. Blood. 2015;125(15):2323–30.
35. Herrlinger U, Schabet M, Brugger W, Kortmann R-D, Küker W, Deckert M, et al. German Cancer Society Neuro-Oncology Working Group NOA-03 multicenter trial of single-agent high-dose methotrexate for primary central nervous system lymphoma. Ann Neurol. 2002;51(2):247–52.
36. Batchelor T, Carson K, O'Neill A, Grossman SA, Alavi J, New P, et al. Treatment of primary CNS lymphoma with methotrexate and deferred radiotherapy: a report of NABTT 96-07. J Clin Oncol. 2003;21(6):1044–9.
37. Ferreri AJM, Cwynarski K, Pulczynski E, Ponzoni M, Deckert M, Politi LS, et al. Chemoimmunotherapy with methotrexate, cytarabine, thiotepa, and rituximab (MATRix regimen) in patients with primary CNS lymphoma: results of the first randomisation of the International Extranodal Lymphoma Study Group-32 (IELSG32) phase 2 trial. Lancet Haematol. 2016;3(5):e217–27.
38. Ferreri AJM, Cwynarski K, Pulczynski E, Fox CP, Schorb E, La Rosée P, et al. Whole-brain radiotherapy or autologous stem-cell transplantation as consolidation strategies after high-dose methotrexate-based chemoimmunotherapy in patients with primary CNS lymphoma: results of the second randomisation of the International Extranodal Lymphoma Study Group-32 phase 2 trial. Lancet Haematol. 2017;4(11):e510–23.
39. Houillier C, Taillandier L, Dureau S, Lamy T, Laadhari M, Chinot O, et al. Radiotherapy or autologous stem-cell transplantation for primary CNS lymphoma in patients 60 years of age and younger: results of the intergroup ANOCEF-GOELAMS randomized phase II PRECIS study. J Clin Oncol. 2019;37(10):823–33.
40. Rubenstein JL, Hsi ED, Johnson JL, Jung S-H, Nakashima MO, Grant B, et al. Intensive chemotherapy and immunotherapy in patients with newly diagnosed primary CNS lymphoma: CALGB 50202 (Alliance 50202). J Clin Oncol. 2013;31(25):3061–8.
41. Weisenburger DD, Savage KJ, Harris NL, Gascoyne RD, Jaffe ES, MacLennan KA, et al. Peripheral T-cell lymphoma, not otherwise specified: a report of 340 cases from the International Peripheral T-cell Lymphoma Project. Blood. 2011;117(12):3402–8.
42. ten Berge RL, de Bruin PC, Oudejans JJ, Ossenkoppele GJ, van der Valk P, Meijer CJLM. ALK-negative anaplastic large-cell lymphoma demonstrates similar poor prognosis to peripheral T-cell lymphoma, unspecified. Histopathology. 2003;43(5):462–9.
43. Gascoyne RD, Aoun P, Wu D, Chhanabhai M, Skinnider BF, Greiner TC, et al. Prognostic significance of anaplastic lymphoma kinase (ALK) protein expression in adults with anaplastic large cell lymphoma. Blood. 1999;93(11):3913–21.

44. Suzuki R, Kagami Y, Takeuchi K, Kami M, Okamoto M, Ichinohasama R, et al. Prognostic significance of CD56 expression for ALK-positive and ALK-negative anaplastic large-cell lymphoma of T/null cell phenotype. Blood. 2000;96(9):2993–3000.
45. Horwitz S, O'Connor OA, Pro B, Illidge T, Fanale M, Advani R, et al. Brentuximab vedotin with chemotherapy for CD30-positive peripheral T-cell lymphoma (ECHELON-2): a global, double-blind, randomised, phase 3 trial. Lancet. 2019;393(10168):229–40.
46. Blystad AK, Enblad G, Kvaløy S, Berglund A, Delabie J, Holte H, et al. High-dose therapy with autologous stem cell transplantation in patients with peripheral T cell lymphomas. Bone Marrow Transplant. 2001;27(7):711–6.
47. Feyler S, Prince HM, Pearce R, Towlson K, Nivison-Smith I, Schey S, et al. The role of high-dose therapy and stem cell rescue in the management of T-cell malignant lymphomas: a BSBMT and ABMTRR study. Bone Marrow Transplant. 2007;40(5):443–50.
48. Jantunen E, Wiklund T, Juvonen E, Putkonen M, Lehtinen T, Kuittinen O, et al. Autologous stem cell transplantation in adult patients with peripheral T-cell lymphoma: a nation-wide survey. Bone Marrow Transplant. 2004;33(4):405–10.
49. Li Y-X, Yao B, Jin J, Wang W-H, Liu Y-P, Song Y-W, et al. Radiotherapy as primary treatment for stage IE and IIE nasal natural killer/T-cell lymphoma. JCO. 2006;24(1):181–9.
50. Kim SJ, Kim K, Kim BS, Kim CY, Suh C, Huh J, et al. Phase II trial of concurrent radiation and weekly cisplatin followed by VIPD chemotherapy in newly diagnosed, stage IE to IIE, nasal, extranodal NK/T-cell lymphoma: consortium for improving survival of lymphoma study. J Clin Oncol. 2009;27(35):6027–32.
51. Jiang M, Zhang H, Jiang Y, Yang Q, Xie L, Liu W, et al. Phase 2 trial of "sandwich" L-asparaginase, vincristine, and prednisone chemotherapy with radiotherapy in newly diagnosed, stage IE to IIE, nasal type, extranodal natural killer/T-cell lymphoma. Cancer. 2012;118(13):3294–301.
52. Wang L, Wang Z, Chen X, Li Y, Wang K, Xia Y, et al. First-line combination of gemcitabine, oxaliplatin, and L-asparaginase (GELOX) followed by involved-field radiation therapy for patients with stage IE/IIE extranodal natural killer/T-cell lymphoma. Cancer. 2013;119(2):348–55.
53. Kwong Y-L, Kim WS, Lim ST, Kim SJ, Tang T, Tse E, et al. SMILE for natural killer/T-cell lymphoma: analysis of safety and efficacy from the Asia Lymphoma Study Group. Blood. 2012;120(15):2973–80.

Radiology of Non-Hodgkin Lymphoma

4

Suman Kumar Ankathi and Nilendu C. Purandare

Contents

S. K. Ankathi
Department of Radiology, Tata Memorial Hospital, Homi Bhabha National Institute,
Mumbai, India

N. C. Purandare (✉)
Department of Nuclear Medicine, Tata Memorial Hospital, Homi Bhabha National Institute,
Mumbai, India

© The Author(s), under exclusive license to Springer Nature Switzerland AG 2021
A. Agrawal et al. (eds.), *PET/CT in Non-Hodgkin Lymphoma*, Clinicians' Guides
to Radionuclide Hybrid Imaging, https://doi.org/10.1007/978-3-030-79007-3_4

4.1   Introduction

Lymphomas affect the lymphoid system and comprise a heterogeneous group of diseases with variable presentation. Diagnostic imaging with Ultrasonography (USG), Computerized Tomography (CT), and Magnetic Resonance Imaging (MRI) provides crucial information for staging and response assessment in patients with lymphoma. This review describes the imaging features of the nodal lymphoma and common extranodal sites of involvement. Summary of multimodality imaging features is described in Table 4.1.

4.2   Nodal Lymphoma

Lymph nodes are the only site of involvement in classic form of Hodgkin's Lymphoma (HL) and low grade Non-Hodgkins lymphoma (NHL). Lymphadenopathy is the most common manifestation of HL with infrequent involvement of extranodal sites (up to 15%). The supradiaphragmatic nodes are involved in 60–68% of patients with HL [1, 2].

The mesenteric and retroperitoneal nodes are more commonly involved in NHL than in HL. In NHL the lymph nodes are markedly enlarged, noncontiguous and frequently associated with extranodal involvement [3, 4].

Table 4.1 Summary of multimodality imaging features of nodal and extranodal sites of lymphomatous involvement

Organ involved	USG	CT	MRI
Nodes	– Conglomerated homogenously hypoechoic lobulated masses – Loss of echogenic hilum with "**pseudocystic**" appearance – Increase in peripheral and central vascularity on color Doppler	NCCT – Enlarged nodes(>10 mm) – Homogenous density CECT – Homogenous enhancement – Cystic changes or necrosis – Encasement of vessels	T1 – Intermediate signal T2/STIR – High signal T1 + c – Homogenous enhancement
Bowel	– Hypoechoic circumferential transmural thickening giving target like appearance – Aneurysmal dilatation of the lumen and intussusception	– Stomach: exophytic submucosal lesion with central ulceration giving typical "**bull's eye**" appearance – Bowel: Diffuse bowel wall thickening or multiple nodular filling defects or aneurysmal bowel dilatation without upstream dilatation	T1 – Homogeneous intermediate signal intensity T2 – Heterogeneous increased signal intensity T1 + c – Mild to moderate homogenous enhancement

Table 4.1 (continued)

Organ involved	USG	CT	MRI
Liver	– Hepatomegaly with homogenously hypoechoic appearance diffusely involving the liver – Focal discrete lesions well defined, homogeneous, markedly hypoechoic or anechoic masses with no posterior acoustic enhancement – The hypoechoic appearance of lymphoma may mimic a hepatic abscess	– Discrete focal liver mass/ Multiple lesions/diffuse infiltrating disease NCCT – Soft tissue attenuation – Necrosis or hemorrhage – Calcification rare CECT – Hypo enhancement to liver parenchyma in all phases – Rim enhancement – Unaffected vessels coursing through mass – Associated splenomegaly and periportal nodal masses	T1 Hypo- or isointense to liver T2 – Moderately hyperintense to liver – Target appearance with hyperintense center and hypointense periphery T1 + c – Target appearance with peripheral enhancement – Hypoenhancing lesions DWI – Restricted diffusion
Spleen	– Massive splenomegaly – Hypoechoic nodules with internal vascularity	– Lower attenuation than adjacent normal splenic parenchyma with minimal or no enhancement	T1 – Low to intermediate signal nodules T2 – Mild to moderately hyperintense T1 + c – Hypoenhancing nodules in delayed phase
Bone	X ray – Lytic, sclerotic, or mixed – Wide zone of transition – Aggressive periosteal reaction – Lesion with extraosseous soft tissue mass	CT – Depicts cortical destruction – Extraosseous soft tissue mass with relative reservation of cortex	T1 – Low marrow signal T2/STIR – High marrow signal DWI – Restricted diffusion T1 + c – Homogenous post contrast enhancement
Lung	– Pleural effusion	– Multiple ill-defined solid or ground glass nodules or masses – Nodules with or without cavitation – Consolidation with air bronchograms, and interlobular – Septal thickening – Direct extension from the adjacent hilar lymph nodes	–

(continued)

Table 4.1 (continued)

Organ involved	USG	CT	MRI
CNS		NCCT – Iso- or hyperdense lesions CECT – Homogenous marked enhancement	T1 – Hypo- or isointense T2 – Hypointense to gray matter DWI – Restricted diffusion T1 + C – Homogeneous intense enhancement. – Ring enhancement MR Spectroscopy – Elevated lipid peaks and high Cho/Cr ratios
Renal	– Solitary or multiple focal hypoechoic masses	NCCT – Solitary/Multiple focal masses/diffuse infiltration in the kidney with slightly higher attenuation than that of the surrounding parenchyma CECT – Homogeneous masses with lower attenuation as compared to the renal cortex	T1 – Hypointense T2 – Hypo to isointense to renal cortex T1 + c – Hypoenhancing masses
Cutaneous	– Soft tissue thickening, infiltration or a mass	– Soft tissue thickening, infiltration or a mass with post contrast enhancement	–

DWI Diffusion-weighted imaging, *STIR* Short tau inversion recovery, *NCCT* Non-contrast enhanced CT, *CECT* Contrast enhanced CT

Ultrasonography (USG) and Computed Tomography (CT) help in the accurate assessment of involved lymph nodes.

4.2.1 USG Features

USG has a major role in initial assessment of the clinically palpable LNs and help in guided biopsies. However, it is not a sensitive modality for staging and assessing deep seated lymph nodes of mediastinum and retroperitoneum. Normal and reactive nodes often have an elongated shape and tend to be hypoechoic as compared to adjacent skeletal muscles with echogenic fatty hilum (Fig. 4.1a). On gray scale

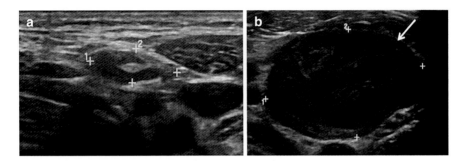

Fig. 4.1 Nodal Lymphoma (Ultrasonography). (**a**) Gray scale ultrasonography reveals a well-defined oblong lymph node with maintained fatty hilum (arrow)-normal appearance. (**b**) Enlarged rounded hypoechoic heterogenous node (arrow) suggestive of lymphomatous involvement (arrow)

USG the enlarged lymphomatous nodes appear as rounded, lobulated masses (Fig. 4.1b) which are homogenously hypoechoic with loss of echogenic hilum giving a "pseudocystic" appearance. On color Doppler, lymphomatous nodes usually show increase in peripheral and central vascularity. However, these features are nonspecific for lymphoma [5–7].

4.2.2   CT

Recognition of lymph node involvement in lymphoma using CT is based entirely on size criteria. The short axis diameter of LNs greater than 1 cm is generally considered as enlarged on CT. On CT the involved lymphnodes are enlarged and of homogenous density (Fig. 4.2). Minimally enlarged discrete nodes tend to have regular borders with homogenous enhancement after administration of IV contrast [6].

4.3   Extranodal Lymphoma

Extranodal involvement may represent a primary manifestation or dissemination of systemic disease. Extranodal involvement is more common in NHL than in HL. CT is the preferred modality, particularly in evaluating hepatic lymphoma and in diagnosing gastrointestinal and renal lymphoma [8, 9].

4.4   Gastrointestinal Lymphoma

Gastointestinal tract is the most common extranodal site of involvement in NHL. Primary GI lymphoma affects stomach, small intestine, and colon in order of decreasing frequency with esophagus involved rarely.

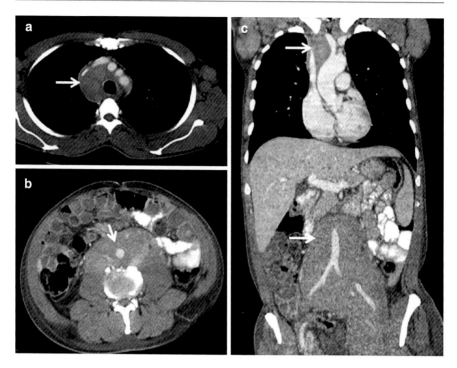

Fig. 4.2 Nodal Lymphoma (CT scan). Axial CECT image of Thorax (**a**) shows enlarged mediastinal nodes (arrow) encasing trachea and displacing branches of Aorta. Axial CECT of Abdomen
(**b**) shows a large conglomerated retroperitoneal nodal mass (arrow) in the paraaortic region
extending up to the external iliac vessels. It is causes compression of the infrarenal IVC without
any significant luminal narrowing of the aorta or its branches. Coronal reformatted Image of thorax
and abdomen (**c**) shows supra and infra diaphragmatic nodal masses

4.4.1 USG Features

On USG these tumors are hypoechoic and most commonly demonstrate circumferential transmural wall thickening giving target like appearance. Other patterns may
be seen, such as segmental, nodular, and bulky tumor. Aneurysmal dilatation of the
lumen and intussusception may also be seen on USG [10, 11].

4.4.2 CT Features

Gastric lymphoma has varied appearance on CT images. Focal or diffuse nodular
thickening of gastric rugae with loss of normal wall layering pattern is best depicted
with distension by negative oral contrast agents (Fig. 4.3). The ulcerative form may
present as exophytic submucosal lesion with central ulceration giving typical "bull's
eye" appearance.

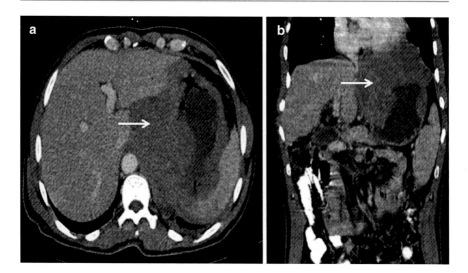

Fig. 4.3 Gastric lymphoma. Axial (**a**) and coronal (**b**) reformatted section of contrast enhanced CT scan shows an ill-defined heterogeneously enhancing soft tissue (arrows) mass arising from the fundus and body of stomach along both lesser and greater curvatures. It is also seen to involve most of the left hemidiaphragm, invading into adjacent lung parenchyma

Primary small bowel lymphoma tends to arise in terminal ileum. It may present as diffuse bowel wall thickening or multiple nodular filling defects or aneurysmal bowel dilatation without upstream dilatation.

Colonic lymphoma is rare, more commonly seen with inflammatory bowel diseases. CT may show a diffuse colonic long segment wall thickening with loss of haustra with associated nodal masses [6, 12].

4.5 Liver

Hepatic lymphoma commonly occurs secondary to the systemic lymphoma in both HL and in NHL and indicates advanced disease. Primary hepatic lymphoma is very rare, usually of NHL large cell type. Hepatic involvement is more frequently associated with splenic involvement [13].

4.5.1 USG Features

Hepatomegaly with homogenously hypoechoic appearance diffusely involving the liver is commonly seen however, is a nonspecific feature. Focal discrete lesions usually present as well defined, homogeneous, markedly hypoechoic or anechoic masses with no posterior acoustic enhancement. The hypoechoic appearance of lymphoma may mimic an hepatic abscess. Presence of a thick wall with septations and mobile internal echoes and heterogenous appearance favor diagnosis of abscess. Associated periportal lymph node involvement is commonly seen [13–15].

4.5.2 CT Features

Diffuse liver infiltration presenting as hepatomegaly with homogenous appearance is more common than multiple discrete hepatic masses (Fig. 4.4). Multiple discrete lesions are homogenously hypodense with minimal to noenhancement on CECT. Patchy or rim enhancement is seen in few cases. However, multiple vascular channels are often seen coursing through the lesion which has been referred to as the "vessel penetration sign." HL manifests as miliary lesions (<1 cm in diameter) which can mimic fungal abscesses which show typical rim enhancement pattern. Mixed infiltrative and nodular pattern of hepatic involvement can also be seen resulting in multiple hypoenhancing nodules in the background of diffuse hepatic enlargement. Periportal spread of lymphoma can manifest as periportal soft tissue cuffing or ill-defined periportal mass. More commonly juxta-hilar mass is seen tracking along biliary radicals and portal tracts. On CT these masses are homogeneously hypodense and encase the portal vessels without occluding them [8, 13, 16].

4.6 Spleen

Lymphoma is the most common malignancy affecting the spleen and maybe primary or secondary.

Spleen is usually considered to be a "nodal organ" in Hodgkin disease and an extranodal organ in non-Hodgkin lymphoma. Splenic involvement is typically diffuse, and only a small minority of cases manifest with nodules larger than 1 cm in

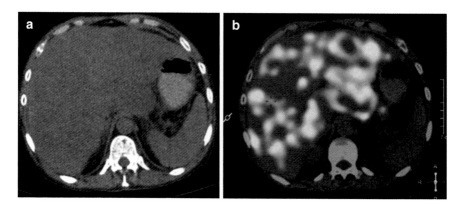

Fig. 4.4 Liver lymphoma. Axial non-contrast CT (**a**) of abdomen shows diffusely enlarged liver with no focal abnormality. On fused FDG PET/CT axial image (**b**) shows multiple foci of abnormal FDG uptake noted throughout the liver

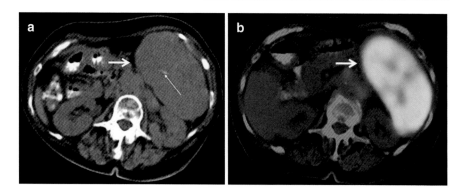

Fig. 4.5 Splenic lymphoma. Axial non-contrast CT (**a**) of abdomen shows diffusely enlarged spleen (arrow) with calcific foci within in the parenchyma (thin arrow). On fused FDG PET/CT axial image (**b**) enlarged spleen shows diffuse increased abnormal FDG uptake (arrow)

diameter. Marked splenomegaly with homogenous enlargement almost always indicates infiltration, however is not specific. USG is more sensitive as compared to CT in detecting splenic nodules which are hypoechoic with internal vascularity. Nodules are characteristically hypoechoic on USG. On CT, they demonstrate lower attenuation than adjacent normal splenic parenchyma with minimal or noenhancement on CECT [8, 17] (Fig. 4.5).

4.7 Pulmonary Lymphoma

Lung parenchymal involvement is more common in HL than NHL and occurs as part of disseminated HL. Primary pulmonary lymphoma without evidence of significant nodal disease is more common in NHL. Pulmonary parenchymal involvement in lymphoma exhibits diverse patterns of abnormality on CT scan. Various manifestations of pulmonary involvement include direct extension from the adjacent hilar lymph nodes, solitary or multiple discrete or confluent nodules forming conglomerate masses, nodules with or without cavitation, consolidation with air bronchograms and reticular patterns with interlobular septal thickening (Fig. 4.6). Pleural effusions seen in association with pulmonary lymphoma tend to be reactive, can be due to lymphatic obstruction and rarely contain malignant cells [18, 19].

4.8 Bone

Primary lymphoma of bone is rare, comprising<1% of all lymphomas and is predominantly of NHL type. Lymphoma can involve bone marrow, cortical bone or both and also extend outside the bone.

Radiographic manifestation of osseous lymphoma is variable and nonspecific. The radiographic pattern can be normal, predominantly lytic, sclerotic, or mixed

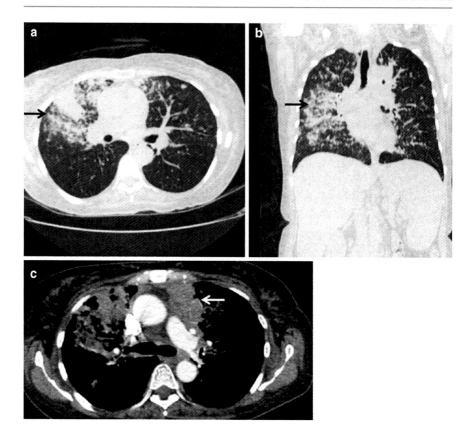

Fig. 4.6 Pulmonary lymphoma. CT Thorax in a known case of low Grade NHL. Axial (**a**) and coronal reformatted section (**b**) of thorax in lung window confluent nodular opacities with surrounding ground glass opacities and interstitial nodular septal thickening seen scattered in both lungs (arrow). Axial section of CECT (**c**) shows of anterior mediastinal mass (arrow). Histopathology showed follicular lymphoma (with diffuse pattern of involvement)

lytic sclerotic. When visible on plain radiographs osseous lymphoma appears as a solitary lytic lesion in the metadiaphyseal region with permeative or moth-eaten pattern of destruction and aggressive periosteal reaction. There may be associated with cortical destruction and extraosseous soft tissue masses (Fig. 4.7). The diffusely sclerotic pattern of the lesions is more frequently seen in Hodgkin's lymphoma. Diffuse sclerosis may be related to fibrosis and can develop following chemotherapy or radiation.

MRI is excellent for evaluation of bone marrow affected by lymphoma and depiction of soft tissue masses. Marrow involvement can be multifocal or diffuse. On T1W images lymphoma within bone marrow is of low signal intensity (relative to adjacent muscle) and gives high signal on T2W and short tau inversion recovery (STIR) sequences. Extraosseous soft tissue masses are of similar signal intensity to the marrow lesion with diffuse andhomogeneous postcontrast enhancement.

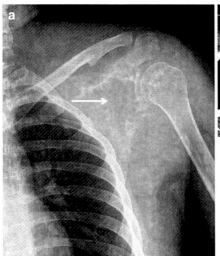
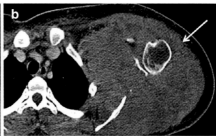

Fig. 4.7 Osseous lymphoma. Plain radiograph (**a**) of left shoulder reveals lytic lesion involving the body of left scapula (arrow) with a large extraosseous soft tissue component. Axial CECT image (**b**) of the left shoulder reveals lysis of the left scapula blade with an associated soft tissue mass infiltrating the adjacent muscles (arrow)

Extraosseous extension of the tumor without cortical destruction is visualized well on MR imaging [20, 21].

4.9   Primary CNS Lymphoma (PCNSL)

Primary CNS lymphoma is rare and occurs almost exclusively within the brain and spinal cord is very rarely involved. Lesions predominantly occur within the cerebral white matter close to the corpus callosum. A butterfly distribution with spread across the corpus callosum seen in lymphoma can mimic diagnosis of butterfly glioma. Posterior fossa may also be involved and can be multifocal in 20% of the cases.

4.9.1   MRI Features

The appearance of intracerebral lymphoma on MRI reflects high cellularity and low water content. On MR imaging the lesions tend to be isointense or low intensity to brain on T1- and T2 weighted images with restricted diffusion and intense enhancement on post-contrast T1W sequences. The lesions appear heterogeneous with peripheral rim enhancement and necrotic center in immunocompromised patients, which may be difficult to differentiate from cerebral abscess. Both lesions show restricted diffusion on DWI MRI (Fig. 4.8). Thin rim of T2 hypointensity may favor a diagnosis of cerebral abscess rather than lymphoma [3, 22].

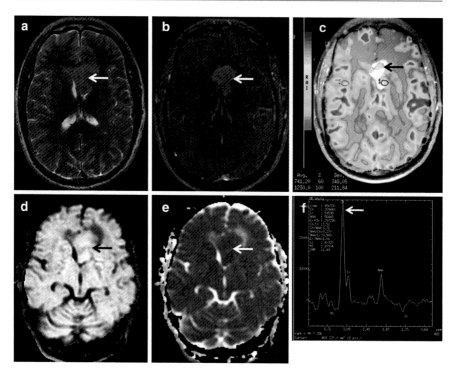

Fig. 4.8 Primary CNS lymphoma. Axial T2W image (**a**) shows iso to hypointense mass lesion in the genu and body of corpus callosum (arrow). Postgadolinium contrast T1W image (**b**) shows homogenous enhancement in the lesion (arrow). Perfusion MRI (**c**) shows low perfusion in the lesion on the relative cerebral blood volume color map (arrow). Diffusion-weighted imaging (**d**) shows high signal intensity in the lesion (arrow) with a corresponding low signal intensity on the apparent diffusion coefficient map (**e**), suggesting restricted diffusion. MR spectroscopy (**f**) shows elevated choline (arrow) with a choline: creatinine ratio 6

4.10   Other Sites

The most common site for extranodal involvement by diffuse large B-cell lymphoma is Waldeyer ring (i.e., lingual, palatine, and nasopharyngeal tonsils). Presence of necrosis within nodes and the absence of distant nodal or extranodal disease should suggest squamous cell carcinoma rather than lymphoproliferative disease [22]. Lymphoma is the most common testicular malignancy in men older than 60 years. Imaging is primarily by ultrasound and follicular lymphoma can present as either diffuse hypoechoic infiltrative mass or solitary discretemasses [12] (Fig. 4.9).The skin is the second most common site of extranodal involvement of

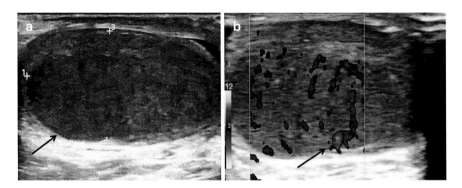

Fig. 4.9 Testicular lymphoma. Gray scale Ultrasound (**a**) of the scrotum demonstrates an enlarged diffusely heterogenous left testis with striated appearance (arrow). Color Doppler ultrasound (**b**) reveals increased vascularity in left testis

NHS after GIT. Primary cutaneous lymphoma is classified as either cutaneous T cell lymphoma or cutaneous B-cell lymphoma. Imaging features of cutaneous lymphoma are nonspecific and include soft tissue thickening, infiltration or a mass and can affect any part of the body with or without localized or diffuse lymphadenopathy [20] (Fig. 4.10). Involvement of the kidneys in lymphoma is usually late and is seen in the presence of disseminated disease. Both solitary and multiple focal masses and diffuse infiltration in the kidney which are hypoenhancing on CECT as compared to the renal cortex have been described (Fig. 4.11).

4.11   Response Evaluation

The Lugano classification represents a major change from the Ann Arbor staging system and the International Working Group criteria for response assessment. The goal of Lugano classification is simplification and standardization of response assessment and reporting. It also addresses the role of FDG PET CT for staging and interim treatment response assessment. The new response criteria using CT are as follows:

Complete radiological response—all nodes reduced to <1.5 cm in longest diameter. Complete disappearance of radiological evidence of disease.

Partial response—50% or greater decrease in disease burden.

Stable disease—less than 50% decrease in disease burden.

Progressive disease—new or increased adenopathy or new extranodal lymphoma [6].

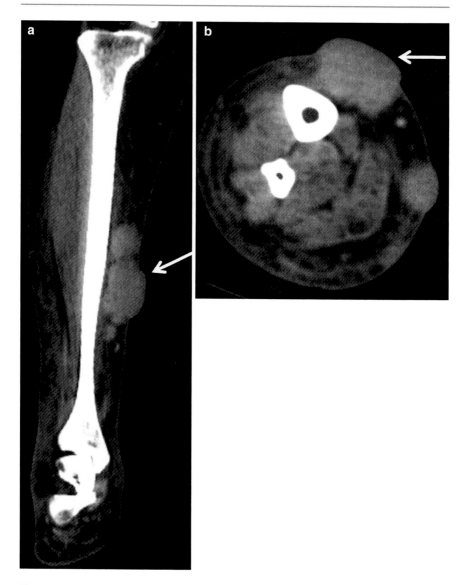

Fig. 4.10 Cutaneous lymphoma. Coronal reformatted (**a**) and axial (**b**) contrast enhanced CT in a case of primary cutaneous lymphoma, shows enhancing subcutaneous soft tissue deposits (arrows) noted in right leg

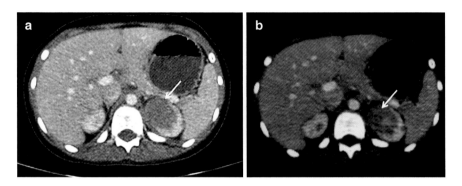

Fig. 4.11   Renal lymphoma. Axial CECT of abdomen at the level of kidneys (**a**) shows a well-defined hypodense lesion arising from the upper pole of the left kidney (arrow). Fused PET/CT image (**b**) show marked increase in tracer uptake with SUV max of 6.5 (arrow) in the left renal upper pole lesion

References

1. Gossmann A, Eich HT, Engert A, et al. CT and MR imaging in Hodgkin's disease–present and future. Eur J Haematol. 2005;75:83–9.
2. Husband J, Reznek RH, Husband JE. Imaging in oncology. Boca Raton: CRC Press; 2016.
3. Vinnicombe M.R.C.P., F.R.C.R. SJ, Reznek M.D. RH, Rohatiner M.D. A. Hematologic malignancy: the lymphomas. In: Silverman M.D. PM, ed.; 2012:531–553.
4. Reznek RH, Richards MA. The radiology of lymphoma. Baillieres Clin Haematol. 1987;1(1):77–107.
5. Ahuja AT, Ying M. Sonographic evaluation of cervical lymph nodes. Am J Roentgenol. 2005;184:1691–9.
6. Johnson SA, Kumar A, Matasar MJ, Schöder H, Rademaker J. Imaging for staging and response assessment in lymphoma. Radiology. 2015;276:323–38.
7. Oscier D, Dearden C, Eren E, et al. Guidelines on the diagnosis, investigation and management of chronic lymphocytic leukaemia. Br J Haematol. 2012;159:541.
8. Guermazi A, Brice P, de Kerviler E, et al. Extranodal Hodgkin disease: Spectrum of disease. Radiographics. 2001;21:161–79.
9. Manzella A, Borba-Filho P, D'Ippolito G, Farias M. Abdominal manifestations of lymphoma: spectrum of imaging features. ISRN Radiol. 2013;2013:483069.
10. Goerg C, Schwerk WB, Goerg K. Gastrointestinal lymphoma: sonographic findings in 54 patients. Am J Roentgenol. 1990;155:795–8.
11. Ghai S, Pattison J, Ghai S, O'Malley ME, Khalili K, Stephens M. Primary gastrointestinal lymphoma: spectrum of imaging findings with pathologic correlation. Radiographics. 2007;27:1371–88.
12. Thomas AG, Vaidhyanath R, Kirke R, Rajesh A. Extranodal lymphoma from head to toe: part 2, the trunk and extremities. Am J Roentgenol. 2011;197:357–64.

13. Rajesh S, Bansal K, Sureka B, Patidar Y, Bihari C, Arora A. The imaging conundrum of hepatic lymphoma revisited. Insights Imaging. 2015;6:679–92.
14. Carroll BA, Ta HN. The ultrasonic appearance of extranodal abdominal lymphoma. Radiology. 1980;136:419–25.
15. Kim H, Kim KW, Park M-S, Kim H. Lymphoma presenting as an echogenic periportal mass: sonographic findings. J Clin Ultrasound. 2008;36:437–9.
16. Anis M, Irshad A. Imaging of abdominal lymphoma. Radiol Clin North Am. 2008;46:265–85.
17. Bhatia K, Sahdev A, Reznek RH. Lymphoma of the spleen. Semin Ultrasound CT MRI. 2007;28:12–20.
18. Hare SS, Souza CA, Bain G, et al. The radiological spectrum of pulmonary lymphoproliferative disease. Br J Radiol. 2012;85:848–64.
19. Lee W-K, Duddalwar VA, Rouse HC, Lau EWF, Bekhit E, Hennessy OF. Extranodal lymphoma in the thorax: cross-sectional imaging findings. Clin Radiol. 2009;64:542–9.
20. Hwang S. Imaging of lymphoma of the musculoskeletal system. Radiol Clin North Am. 2008;46:379–96.
21. Krishnan A, Shirkhoda A, Tehranzadeh J, Armin AR, Irwin R, Les K. Primary bone lymphoma: radiographic–MR imaging correlation. Radiographics. 2003;23:1371–83.
22. Thomas AG, Vaidhyanath R, Kirke R, Rajesh A. Extranodal lymphoma from head to toe: part 1, the head and spine. Am J Roentgenol. 2011;197:350–6.

PET CT in Non-Hodgkin Lymphoma

5

Archi Agrawal, M. V. Manikandan, Abhishek Uppal, and Venkatesh Rangarajan

Contents

5.1 Introduction

18F-Fluorodeoxyglucose Positron Emission Tomography combined with Computed Tomography (FDG PET/CT) is now the standard imaging modality for staging and assessment of response in all FDG avid Non-Hodgkin Lymphoma (NHL). FDG PET/CT plays a central point in treatment decisions in lymphoma. Most NHLs are FDG avid, viz. diffuse large B-cell lymphoma (DLBCL), Burkitt lymphoma, follicular and mantle cell lymphoma (MCL). But some indolent NHLs like small lymphocytic

A. Agrawal (✉) · M. V. Manikandan · A. Uppal · V. Rangarajan
Department of Nuclear Medicine and Molecular Imaging, Tata Memorial Hospital, Homi Bhabha National Institute, Mumbai, India

lymphoma, chronic lymphocytic leukemia, marginal zone lymphoma show low or variable FDG avidity and thus functional imaging with FDG PET/CT is of limited usefulness [1, 2]. PET CT is the most reliable modality of imaging for assessment of response after completion of therapy. Response assessment criteria in lymphomas have seen multiple transitions, starting from International Working Group criteria (IWG) developed in 1999 [3] to the Response Evaluation Criteria in Lymphoma [4] criteria developed in 2017. The IWG criteria created an entity called "complete remission – unconfirmed" (CRu) based on residual mass after treatment. This led to confusion, as outcomes of patients with complete remission (CR) or partial response (PR) based on CT criteria were similar, as long as there was no FDG avid residual disease. This CRu was abolished in the revised criteria that was published in 2007 called International Harmonization Project (IHP) criteria and was based on metabolic activity of FDG PET/CT [5]. The fallacy of this criterion was that the FDG avidity was defined based on mediastinal blood pool activity. This was rectified by the Deauville criterion which was formulated in 2009 [6]. Finally the Lugano classification in 2014 incorporated both CT and PET/CT into the response assessment criteria and stated that PET/CT be used for all FDG avid histologies using a 5-point Deauville score and CT be used for all non-FDG avid and low-FDG avid histologies [7]. With this background we shall see the role of FDG PET/CT in NHL.

5.2 Staging

Defining the exact extent and location of disease is the crux for providing the correct treatment and in prognosticating the patients. ^{18}F-FDG PET/CT is the standard imaging modality for staging of all FDG avid NHLs (Fig. 5.1). PET/CT has better accuracy for staging of nodal and extranodal sites as compared to CT [8]. PET/CT is better at detecting lymphomatous involvement in small sized nodes and has a higher sensitivity in detection of extranodal involvement as compared to CT (Figs. 5.2 and 5.3). This leads to a change in stage culminating in change in management in up to 25% of the patients [9, 10].

In a large study with 520 patients (59% of these were DLBCL) of NHL, done by Metser et al. and published in 2019, they compared the change in management and outcomes in patients with lymphoma who had undergone CT and PET/CT. PET/CT upstaged 28% of patients with NHL who were classified as limited stage disease on CT. 56% of patients with equivocal findings on CT were correctly classified as advanced-stage disease by PET/CT. The outcomes were better in patients staged by PET/CT. They showed better overall survival in patients with PET/CT guided management [11].

5.2.1 Bulky Disease

Patients with bulky disease receive consolidative external radiotherapy in addition to the chemotherapy [12, 13]. However, there is no clear-cut definition of bulky disease and varies from institution to institution. In our institution 7 cm in the longest dimension is considered as bulky for DLBCL.

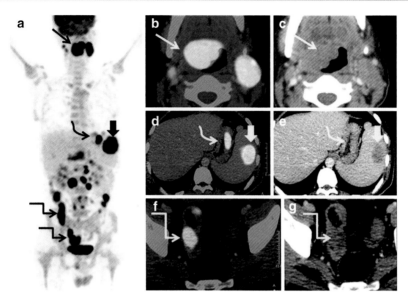

Fig. 5.1 45 years male, a case of Diffuse Large B-cell lymphoma for a staging PET/CT scan. Multiple sites of involvement are noted. MIP and axial PET/CT images show hypermetabolic foci involving left tonsil, vallecula, and base of tongue (arrows). Involvement of stomach (curved arrow), bowel (sharp bent arrow), and spleen (block arrow) is seen

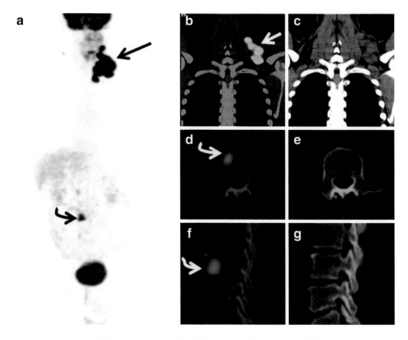

Fig. 5.2 39 years male, NHL for staging PET CT study. MIP and axial PET CT show hypermetabolic left cervical adenopathy (arrow in **a**–**c**). Also seen is focal marrow involvement in L3 vertebral body (curved arrow in **a**, **d**, **f**). The marrow lesion is not evident on the corresponding CT image (**e**, **g**). Thus PET CT has upstaged the disease from stage I to IV

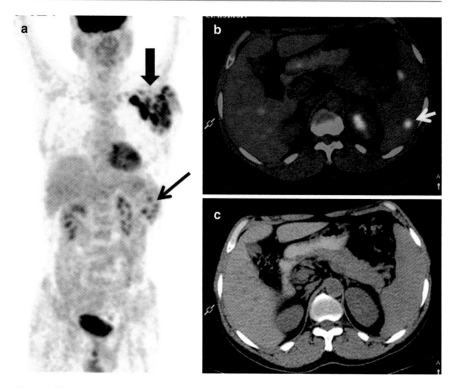

Fig. 5.3 PET CT scan done for staging in a 50 years old male, a case of NHL. MIP and axial PET CT show multiple hypermetabolic left axillary nodes (block arrow in **a**). Tiny hypermetabolic foci are noted in the spleen (arrow in **a, b**). Upstaging of the disease by PET CT from stage I to stage III

5.2.2 Spleen

Splenic involvement on FDG PET CT may either be focal or diffuse. Focal involvement is seen as FDG avid areas in spleen (Fig. 5.4). Splenic uptake 1.5 times higher than the liver uptake, in the absence of diffuse marrow uptake, is the criterion for detection of diffuse spleen involvement (Fig. 5.5) [12]. Diffuse uptake on PET CT can sometimes be associated with reactive changes, similar to that seen in bone marrow. Splenomegaly more than 13 cm is taken as involved by the Lugano classification [7].

5.2.3 Liver

PET CT is better than CT in detection of lymphomatous involvement in the liver. Hepatic involvement is manifested as focal or diffuse uptake on PET CT similar to spleen (Fig. 5.6).

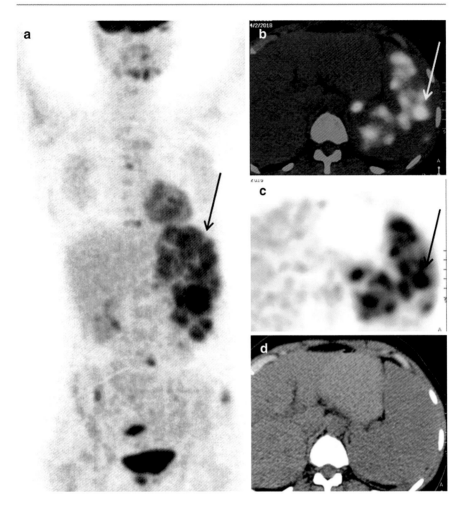

Fig. 5.4 PET CT scan in a case of NHL shows multiple foci of FDG avid lesions in the spleen (arrow)

5.2.4   Bone Marrow

Bone marrow involvement is frequently seen in patients with NHL, particularly DLBCL. PET/CT is a sensitive modality for detection of focal disease in the bone marrow in DLBCL (Fig. 5.7). PET/CT is better than biopsy in detection of large lymphomatous cells in the bone marrow, but PET/CT may miss low-volume disease and small lymphomatous cells in the bone marrow [14–16]. The specificity of detection of bone marrow disease in diffuse hypermetabolic marrow is low as reactive marrow changes may predominate (Figs. 5.8 and 5.9) [14]. Patients who have confirmed marrow involvement on PET CT and bone marrow biopsy have a worse prognosis than patients who have bone marrow involvement only on PET [14, 16].

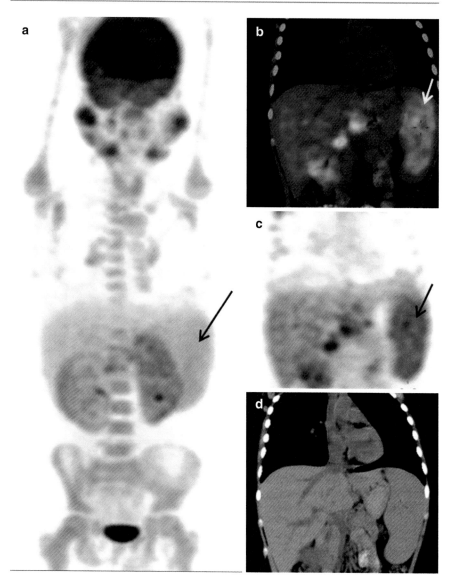

Fig. 5.5 PET CT in a 22 year old, a case of NHL shows diffuse increased FDG uptake in the spleen suggestive of lymphomatous involvement of spleen (arrow)

This is more likely due to large burden of disease. The Lugano classification still recommends a bone marrow biopsy in DLBCL as PET/CT can miss low-volume disease in 10–20% of patients [7, 17–19]. In advanced-stage NHL, if the PET/CT is positive for marrow involvement, a bone marrow biopsy may be avoided. If PET/CT is negative for marrow involvement, then a bone marrow biopsy is indicated [15, 20]. The sensitivity of PET CT in detecting bone marrow disease ranges from 71 to

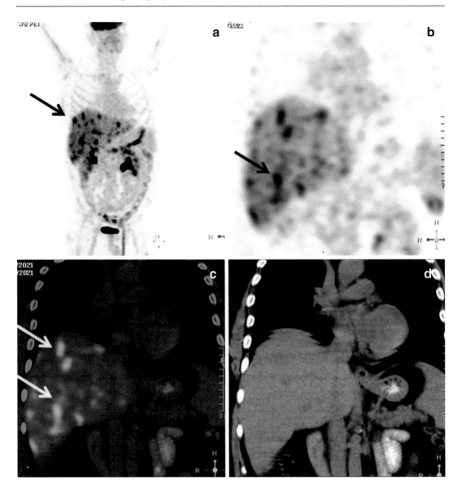

Fig. 5.6 54 year old male, case of relapsed NHL. PET CT study shows multiple FDG avid foci involving the liver (arrows)

95% with a very high specificity of 99–100% [20]. For all other histologies of NHL, a bone marrow biopsy is indicated.

5.3   Response Assessment

Assessment of response for lymphoma has been one of the earliest indications of PET CT. PET/CT is the most reliable imaging modality for response assessment. In aggressive NHL, PET CT is used to assess remission after completion of treatment and to identify patients who have failed the first line treatment. This subset of patients either undergo a follow-up PET CT scan or are considered for second-line or salvage therapy after confirmation of residual disease [21].

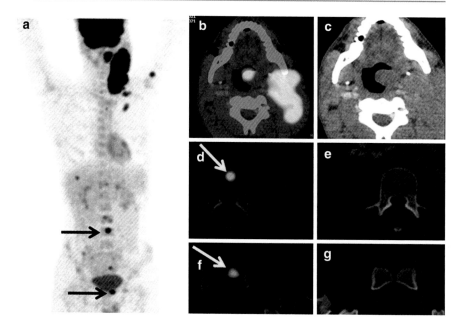

Fig. 5.7 18 year old boy, a case of NHL. MIP and axial PET CT study show focal hypermetabolic marrow lesions in multiple sites; those marked are seen in the lumbar vertebra and left pubic bone

Response assessment can be done early after the start of treatment, usually after completion of 2 or 3 cycles of chemotherapy, when it is called "**interim PET**" or after completion of the chemotherapy regime, which is called as "**End-of-treatment**" response.

5.3.1 Interim PET (i-PET)

i-PET is helpful in assessing the chemosensitivity in aggressive NHL but unlike Hodgkins lymphoma, cannot be routinely used for modification of the treatment regime. A negative i-PET is associated with negative end-of-treatment PET and with good outcomes [22, 23]. But conversely, patients of DLBCL with a positive i-PET are reported to have remission after completion of the R-CHOP regimen (Rituximab-Cyclophosphamide, Hydroxydaunorubicin, Oncovin [Vincristine sulfate], Prednisolone), with overall survival of 92% [23]. Thus though an i-PET has a very high negative predictive value, false-positives can occur and thus treatment modification is rarely done.

5.3.2 Deauville Criteria

Deauville criteria is based on a 5-point scale currently used for response assessment with FDG PET/CT [6] (Table 5.1). A score of 1 and 2 is suggestive of complete metabolic response, both in interim and end-of-treatment response assessment. Here the uptake is less than or equal to the mediastinal blood pool activity (Fig. 5.10).

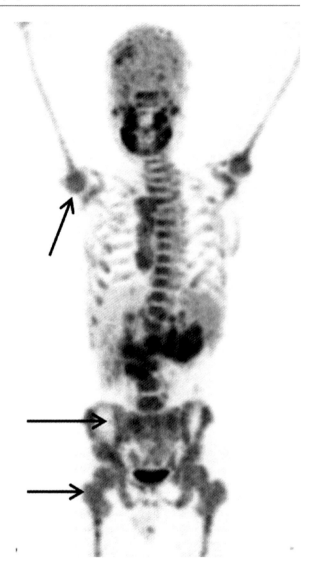

Fig. 5.8 20 year old male, diagnosed case of NHL. PET CT shows intense, diffuse uptake in the marrow of axial and appendicular skeleton, suggestive of bone marrow involvement (arrows)

A score of 3 shows uptake greater than mediastinal uptake, but less than or equal to liver (Fig. 5.11). Most patients with a score of 3 at interim evaluation have good prognosis at the end of therapy in most NHLs [24, 25]. However in the trial setting, especially for trials contemplating de-escalation of the chemotherapy regime, a more judicious approach is recommended in order to avoid under-treatment.

A score of 4 or 5 (uptake more than the liver) at the end-of-treatment represents residual disease, even if there is decrease in the SUV value from the baseline (Fig. 5.12). On interim evaluation, if the uptake has reduced from baseline, it is considered as partial metabolic response and that the disease is sensitive to chemotherapy. However, a score of 4 or 5 with no decrease or increase in uptake from

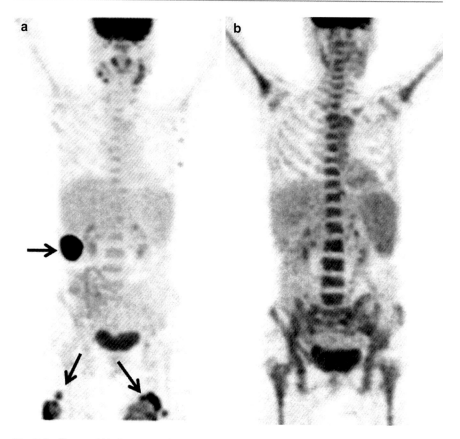

Fig. 5.9 48 year old lady, a case of NHL with subcutaneous lesions. Staging PET CT scan in (**a**) shows cutaneous lesions (arrow). The MIP image on right (**b**) shows diffuse uptake in the marrow due to reactive marrow stimulation post-chemotherapy

Table 5.1 Deauville criteria for response assessment

Deauville criteria for response assessment [6]	
Score	Uptake
1	No uptake
2	Uptake < Mediastinum
3	Uptake > Mediastinum < Liver
4	Uptake moderately higher than liver
5	Uptake markedly higher than liver and/or new lymphomatous lesions

baseline is considered as failure of treatment at both interim and end of therapy evaluation. Same is the scenario if new foci suggestive of lymphomatous involvement are seen.

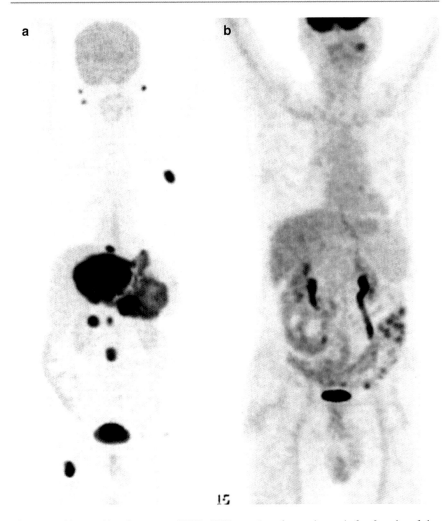

Fig. 5.10 66 year old male, a case of NHL. PET scan done for staging and after 2 cycles of chemotherapy. MIP image shows multiple supra and infradiaphragmatic adenopapthy with bulky nodal mass in the abdomen in (**a**). The post 2# MIP image shows complete metabolic response in (**b**). This is Deauville score 1

5.3.3   End-of-Treatment PET/CT

In aggressive NHL, end-of-treatment PET CT has a very high negative predictive value of 80–100%. The positive predictive value of end-of-treatment PET CT varies from 50 to 100%, meaning that treatment based on a positive PET CT has to be substantiated by a biopsy or a follow-up scan to rule out the possibility of benign/inflammatory etiology [26–28]. Positive PET CT after R-CHOP has a poor prognosis. Consolidative radiotherapy to residual PET positive masses has shown improved outcomes [29–31].

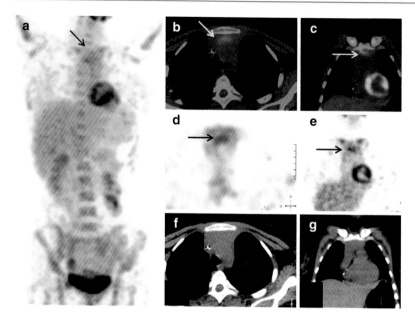

Fig. 5.11 25 year old lady, case of mediastinal B-cell lymphoma. PET scan was done after 3 # of chemotherapy. MIP, axial and coronal images show residual mediastinal mass with FDG uptake equal to the liver (arrows). This is Deauville score 3

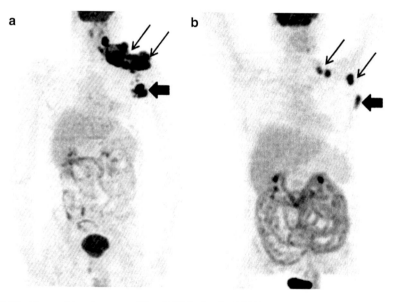

Fig. 5.12 44 year old male, a case of B-cell NHL. Staging PET CT shows multiple conglomerated left supraclavicular nodal mass (arrow), left axillary nodes (arrow), and involvement of scapula (block arrow). Post 6 cycles of chemotherapy PET CT show decrease in size and metabolic activity of the lesions with residual disease. The intensity of FDG uptake is greater than liver, Deauville score 4

5.3.4   Response Assessment After Immunotherapy

With the advent of immune check point inhibitors or the novel immunotherapy, interpreting FDG PET CT has become a challenge. The mechanism of action of these agents leads to different pattern of response which may mimic progression of disease. This is usually transient and is called as pseudo-progression. LYRIC (The Lymphoma Response to Immunomodulatory therapy Criteria) response criteria is a special criteria developed to assess response after immune-based chemotherapy. In pseudo-progression, the imaging findings suggest an increase in size and metabolic activity of the lesions, without any clinical deterioration of the patient. This is called as indeterminate response (IR) in LYRIC criteria and such a response mandates repeat imaging after 12 weeks to differentiate pseudo-progression from true progression of disease [32].

5.4   FDG PET CT for Radiotherapy Planning

Radiotherapy planning with PET CT helps in precise localization of disease and also helps in modifying the target volume. CT is not very useful as it lacks the functional information of PET imaging. PET helps in identifying small areas of residual disease which are metabolically active and CT helps in correct anatomic localization, thus fused PET CT gives the exact metabolic and anatomic information needed for radiotherapy planning [33].

5.5   FDG PET CT in Relapsed NHL

In relapsed aggressive NHL, second-line, high dose chemotherapy is given to induce remission and to facilitate Autologous Stem Cell Transplant (ASCT) if need be. ASCT is a curative method of treatment. Pre-transplant PET CT is an important prognosticator in patients undergoing ASCT [34, 35]. Patients with a negative PET prior to ASCT have better PFS (progression free survival) and OS rates of 87% and 94% as compared to 35% and 67% in patients with positive PET CT study [34].

5.6   FDG PET CT in Surveillance

There is no role of surveillance scan in a treated case of NHL. Follow-up PET CT is associated with false-positive findings in 20% of patients, this leads to unnecessary investigations, radiation burden, biopsies, cost, and patient anxiety [36, 37]. Only when there is a clinical suspicion of disease relapse, a follow-up scan needs to be done. Prudent use of follow-up scan in cases of indolent lymphoma with residual disease may be contemplated.

References

1. Zelenetz AD, Maragulia J, Horwitz SM. Baseline staging evaluation in lymphoma: the role of FDG PET, CT, and bone marrow biopsy. Blood. 2011;118(21):2640.
2. Weiler-Sagie M, Bushelev O, Epelbaum R, et al. (18)F FDG avidity in lymphoma readdressed: a study of 766 patients. J Nucl Med. 2010;51(1):25–30.
3. Cheson BD, Horning SJ, Coiffier B, et al. Report of an international workshop to standardize response criteria for non-Hodgkin's lymphomas. NCI Sponsored International Working Group. J Clin Oncol. 1999;17(4):1244.
4. Younes A, Hilden P, Coiffier B, Hagenbeek A, Salles G, et al. International Working Group consensus response evaluation criteria in lymphoma (RECIL 2017). Ann Oncol. 2017;28(7):1436–47.
5. Cheson BD. The International Harmonization Project for response criteria in lymphoma clinical trials. Hematol Oncol Clin North Am. 2007;21(5):841–54.
6. Meignan M, Gallamini A, Meignan M, Gallamini A, Haioun C. Report on the First International Workshop on Interim-PET-Scan in Lymphoma. Leuk Lymphoma. 2009;50(8):1257–60.
7. Cheson BD, Fisher RI, Barrington SF, et al. Recommendations for initial evaluation, staging, and response assessment of Hodgkin and non-Hodgkin lymphoma: the Lugano classification. J Clin Oncol. 2014;32:3059–68.
8. Cheson BD. Role of functional imaging in the management of lymphoma. J Clin Oncol. 2011;29:1844–54.
9. Raanani P, Shasha Y, Perry C, et al. Is CT scan still necessary for staging in Hodgkin and non-Hodgkin lymphoma patients in the PET/CT era? Ann Oncol. 2006;17:117–22.
10. Le Dortz L, De Guibert S, Bayat S, et al. Diagnostic and prognostic impact of 18F-FDG PET/CT in follicular lymphoma. Eur J Nucl Med Mol Imaging. 2010;37:2307–14.
11. Metser U, Prica A, Hodgson DC, et al. Effect of PET/CT on the management and outcomes of participants with Hodgkin and aggressive non-Hodgkin lymphoma: a multicenter registry. Radiology. 2019;290:488–95.
12. Pfreundschuh M, Christofyllakis K, Altmann B, et al. Radiotherapy to bulky disease PET-negative after immunochemotherapy in elderly DLBCL patients: results of a planned interim analysis of the first 187 patients with bulky disease treated in the OPTIMAL>60 study of the DSHNHL. Hematol Oncol. 2017;35:129–30.
13. Pfreundschuh M, Ho AD, Cavallin-Stahl E, et al. Prognostic significance of maximum tumour (bulk) diameter in young adults with good-prognosis diffuse large-B-cell lymphoma treated with CHOP like chemotherapy with or without rituximab: an exploratory analysis of the MabThera International Trial Group (MInT) study. Lancet Oncol. 2008;9:435–44.
14. Cerci JJ, Györke T, Fanti S, et al. Combined PET and biopsy evidence of marrow involvement improves prognostic prediction in diffuse large B-cell lymphoma. J Nucl Med. 2014;55:1591–7.
15. Khan AB, Barrington SF, Mikhaeel NG, et al. PET-CT staging of DLBCL accurately identifies and provides new insight into the clinical significance of bone marrow involvement. Blood. 2013;122:61–7.
16. Alzahrani M, El-Galaly TC, Hutchings M, et al. The value of routine bone marrow biopsy in patients with diffuse large B-cell lymphoma staged with PET/CT: a Danish-Canadian study. Ann Oncol. 2016;27:1095–9.
17. Carr R, Barrington SF, Madan B, et al. Detection of lymphoma in bone marrow by whole-body positron emission tomography. Blood. 1998;91:3340–6.
18. Pelosi E, Penna D, Douroukas A, et al. Bone marrow disease detection with FDG-PET/CT and bone marrow biopsy during the staging of malignant lymphoma: results from a large multicentre study. Q J Nucl Med Mol Imaging. 2011;55:469–75.
19. Berthet L, Cochet A, Kanoun S, et al. In newly diagnosed diffuse large B-cell lymphoma, determination of bone marrow involvement with 18F-FDG PET/CT provides better diagnostic performance and prognostic stratification than does biopsy. J Nucl Med. 2013;54:1244–50.

20. Adams HJ, Kwee TC, de Keizer B, et al. FDG PET/CT for the detection of bone marrow involvement in diffuse large B-cell lymphoma: systematic review and meta-analysis. Eur J Nucl Med Mol Imaging. 2014;41:565–74.
21. Barrington SF, Trotman J. The role of PET in the first-line treatment of the most common subtypes of non-Hodgkin lymphoma. Lancet Haematol. 2021;8(1):e80–93.
22. Mamot C, Klingbiel D, Hitz F, et al. Final results of a prospective evaluation of the predictive value of interim positron emission tomography in patients with diffuse large B-cell lymphoma treated with R-CHOP-14 (SAKK 38/07). J Clin Oncol. 2015;33:2523–9.
23. Carr R, Fanti S, Paez D, et al. Prospective international cohort study demonstrates inability of interim PET to predict treatment failure in diffuse large B-cell lymphoma. J Nucl Med. 2014;55:1936–44.
24. Pregno P, Chiapella A, Bello M, et al. Interim 18-FDG-PET/CT failed to predict the outcome in diffuse large B-cell lymphoma patients treated at the diagnosis with rituximab-CHOP. Blood. 2012;119:2066–73.
25. Dupuis J, Berriolo-Riedinger A, Julian A, et al. Impact of [(18)F]fluorodeoxyglucose positron emission tomography response evaluation in patients with high-tumor burden follicular lymphoma treated with immunochemotherapy: a prospective study from the Groupe d'Etudes des Lymphomes de l'Adulte and GOELAMS. J Clin Oncol. 2012;30:4317–22.
26. Cashen AF, Dehdashti F, Luo J, et al. 18F-FDG PET/CT for early response assessment in diffuse large B-cell lymphoma: poor predictive value of international harmonization project interpretation. J Nucl Med. 2011;52:386–92.
27. Micallef IN, Maurer MJ, Wiseman GA, et al. Epratuzumab with rituximab, cyclophosphamide, doxorubicin, vincristine, and prednisone chemotherapy in patients with previously untreated diffuse large B-cell lymphoma. Blood. 2011;118:4053–61.
28. Mikhaeel NG, Timothy AR, Hain SF, et al. 18-FDG-PET for the assessment of residual masses on CT following treatment of lymphomas. Ann Oncol. 2000;11:147–50.
29. Phan J, Mazloom A, Medeiros LJ, et al. Benefit of consolidative radiation therapy in patients with diffuse large B-cell lymphoma treated with R-CHOP chemotherapy. J Clin Oncol. 2010;28:4170–6.
30. Shi Z, Das S, Okwan-Duodu D, et al. Patterns of failure in advanced stage diffuse large B-cell lymphoma patients after complete response to r-chop immunochemotherapy and the emerging role of on solidative radiation therapy. Int J Radiat Oncol Biol Phys. 2013;86:569–77.
31. Dorth JA, Prosnitz LR, Broadwater G, et al. Impact of consolidation radiation therapy in stage III-IV diffuse large B-cell lymphoma with negative post-chemotherapy radiologic imaging. Int J Radiat Oncol Biol Phys. 2012;84:762–7.
32. Cheson BD, Ansell S, Schwartz L, et al. Refinement of the Lugano classification lymphoma response criteria in the era of immunomodulatory therapy. Blood. 2016;128:2489–96.
33. Terezakis SA, Hunt MA, Kowalski A, et al. [18F]FDG-positron emission tomography coregistration with computed tomography scans for radiation treatment planning of lymphoma and hematologic malignancies. Int J Radiat Oncol Biol Phys. 2011;81:615–22.
34. Derenzini E, Musuraca G, Fanti S, Stefoni V, Tani M, Alinari L, Venturini F, Gandolfi L, Baccarani M, Zinzani PL. Pretransplantation positron emission tomography scan is the main predictor of autologous stem cell transplantation outcome in aggressive B-cell non-Hodgkin lymphoma. Cancer. 2008;113(9):2496–503.
35. Sauter CS, Matasar MJ, Meikle J, Schoder H, Ulaner GA, Migliacci JC, Hilden P, Devlin SM, Zelenetz AD, Moskowitz CH. Prognostic value of FDG-PET prior to autologous stem cell transplantation for relapsed and refractory diffuse large B-cell lymphoma. Blood. 2015;125(16):2579–81.
36. Liedtke M, Hamlin PA, Moskowitz CH, et al. Surveillance imaging during remission identifies a group of patients with more favorable aggressive NHL at time of relapse: a retrospective analysis of a uniformly-treated patient population. Ann Oncol. 2006;17:909–13.
37. Zinzani PL, Stefoni V, Tani M, et al. Role of [18F]fluorodeoxyglucose positron emission tomography scan in the follow-up of lymphoma. J Clin Oncol. 2009;27:1781–7.

PET/CT: Normal Variants, Artefacts and Pitfalls in Non-Hodgkin Lymphoma

6

Ameya D. Puranik and Sneha Shah

Contents

6.1   Introduction

Positron Emission Tomography/Computed Tomography (PET/CT) has stamped its place as the investigation of choice for staging, restaging, response assessment and follow-up of patients with lymphoma. The favourable GLUT (GLUcose-Transporter) receptor expression of the proliferating lymphocytes makes it the most physiological modality for evaluating lymphomas at every step [1]. Multiple other cellular pathways involving infective and inflammatory processes also depend on the GLUT expression mechanism, and hence can pose diagnostic challenge when PET/CT studies for lymphoma are being reported. We tried to document the various artefacts, pitfalls and normal variants on FDG PET/CT which can be kept in mind, in order to avoid false-positive or false-negative results.

A. D. Puranik (✉) · S. Shah
Department of Nuclear Medicine and Molecular Imaging, Tata Memorial Hospital, Homi Bhabha National Institute, Mumbai, India

© The Author(s), under exclusive license to Springer Nature Switzerland AG 2021   71
A. Agrawal et al. (eds.), *PET/CT in Non-Hodgkin Lymphoma*, Clinicians' Guides to Radionuclide Hybrid Imaging, https://doi.org/10.1007/978-3-030-79007-3_6

6.2   FDG Uptake in Lymphoma

FDG is transported into cells by glucose transporters and is phosphorylated once inside the cell. However, the rate of dephosphorylation of FDG-6-phosphate is much slower than that of glucose-6-phosphate, so that 'FDG' effectively accumulates inside the cell in proportion to the rate of glycolysis. The earliest recommendation for use of FDG PET/CT in lymphomas was formulated under the International Harmonisation Project [2], where in depending upon the intensity of tracer uptake, lymphomas were classified as:

– FDG avid
  1. Diffuse Large B-Cell Lymphoma
  2. Hodgkin's Lymphoma
  3. Mantle Cell Lymphoma
– Variably FDG avid
  1. Other aggressive NHLs
  2. Other indolent NHLs

Table 6.1 gives an overview with regard to intensity of uptake of FDG in various pathological subtypes of lymphoma, based on WHO Classification, in a study of 766 patients [2].

Table 6.1   FDG avidity in different histological subtypes

Histological subtype	FDG avidity
Hodgkin's lymphoma	High
Burkitt's lymphoma	High
Mantle cell lymphoma	High
Anaplastic large T-cell lymphoma	High
Marginal zone lymphoma, nodal	High
Lymphoblastic lymphoma	High
Angioimmunoblastic T-cell lymphoma	High
Plasmacytoma	High
Natural killer T-cell lymphoma	High
Diffuse large B-cell lymphoma	High
Follicular lymphoma Grade 3	High
Follicular lymphoma Grade 1, 2	Low to moderate
Peripheral T-cell lymphoma	Low to moderate
Small lymphocytic lymphoma	Low
Enteropathy type T-cell lymphoma	Low
Marginal zone, splenic	Low
MALT marginal zone	Low
Lymphomatoid papulosis	Low
Cutaneous T-cell lymphoma	Low

6.3   Challenges in Reporting PET/CT Studies

FDG PET/CT helps in staging lymphomas, depending upon the extent of involvement, however variable degree of uptake poses a challenge [3]. Size remains an important limiting factor for localisation of FDG; hence any lesion less than 6–8 mm often shows no FDG uptake, as it falls beyond the resolution of PET scanner. Other technical factors like dose of radiopharmaceutical injected, serum glucose levels, timing of scan acquisition and use of steroids interfere with the concentration of FDG, often yielding false negative results [4].

Apart from this, there are many other factors and variations, from the clinical or imaging perspective which can pose challenges. 'Artefacts' are the findings on the scan which give a false-positive appearance owing to technical issues like improper tracer localisation or retention. 'Variants' are the false-positive interpretations resulting from altered or physiological biodistribution of FDG in the body. This arises because of the biochemical pathways which lead to uptake of FDG at normal sites, and its appearance on the scan mimics that of lymphomatous involvement. 'Pitfalls' are the pathological processes which have the same scan findings as that of lymphoma, and often create a diagnostic dilemma (Fig. 6.1). We, in Table 6.2, have addressed almost all possible sources of misinterpretation, discussed its cause and provided imaging based interpretative pointers to distinguish these from actual lymphomatous involvement.

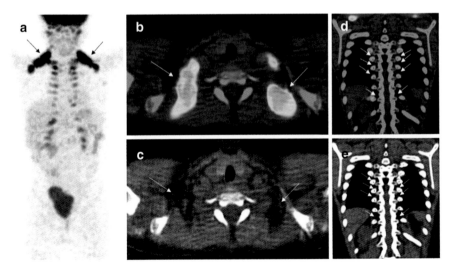

Fig. 6.1 Maximum Intensity Projection (MIP—**a**), axial (**b**—arrow) and coronal (**d**—arrow) show intense FDG uptake in bilateral neck and midline thoracic region, which shows fat-density on CT images (**c**, **e**—arrows). This pattern of uptake is seen in brown adipose tissue

Table 6.2 Variants, artefacts and pitfalls on FDG PET/CT

Normal Variants	Causes	Pointers to Identify
Waldeyer's ring (Fig. 6.2)	Uptake due to the physiological concentration of FDG in macrophages and lymphocytes	Symmetrical uptake Intensity of uptake Uptake will persist even on post-treatment scans
Thymus (Fig. 6.3)	Rebound hyperplasia occurs post-chemotherapy, or is seen normally in infants	CT features of diffuse enlargement with 'inverted V' sign in midline helps differentiate it from lymphoid thymic hyperplasia
Marrow hyperplasia (Fig. 6.4)	In patients who have received chemotherapy or colony stimulating factors, there is hyperstimulation of marrow, resulting in high FDG uptake	Diffuse uniform symmetrical uptake in the entire marrow of appendicular and axial skeleton, with no focal areas of FDG avidity
Bowel uptake (Fig. 6.5)	Physiological FDG uptake is seen either due to FDG secretion into the intestines, or in the lymphoid patches in intestinal mucosa	Focal or diffuse FDG uptake in the bowel loops, with no detectable morphological

Artefacts	Cause	Pointers to identify
Port site retention	Inflammatory reaction increase macrophages and IF factors	Presence of a post—seen as dense object at known sites of port localisation
Injection extravasation (Fig. 6.6)	Focal radionuclide deposition	History of site of injection, swelling, associated pain

Pitfalls	Causes	Pointers to identify
Low grade lymphomas [6] (Fig. 6.7)	Indolent or low grade lymphomas, especially CLL and small lymphocytic lymphoma (SLL) show low or absent GLUT receptor expression, respectively	Multi-station non-necrotic nodal enlargement with contrast enhancement, with or without splenomegaly and marrow uptake; in addition to clinical features of fever, weight loss
Mantle cell lymphoma [7]	Variable avidity reported in literature	Same as above
Follicular lymphoma (FL) [8]	Though classified as lymphoma with high grade uptake, grade 1 and 2 FL typically show low FDG avidity	Same as above
Primary extranodal lymphoma mimicking primary neoplasm (Fig. 6.8)	High grade uptake in a single site with absence of or contiguous nodal involvement	No discrete imaging features to differentiate
Splenic hyperplasia	Diffuse intense FDG uptake in enlarged spleen	Interim scan helpful—lymphomatous splenic involvement shows FDG uptake greater than liver with reduction in uptake after treatment while hyperplasia shows increased uptake but similar to or less than liver with no change in uptake at interim scan It is accompanied by presence of diffuse marrow uptake if associated with haematological dysfunction

Table 6.2 (continued)

Bowel inflammation in Burkitt's lymphoma	Common site of involvement in Burkitt's lymphoma is intestinal loops	Post-chemotherapy, involved bowel loop will show reduction in uptake within the involved lymphatics of bowel but may show uptake in the inflamed mucosal layer
Mesenteric panniculitis (Fig. 6.9)		
Infections and inflammations [9]	Increased GLUT receptor expression in following:	CT features of necrotic nodes, with/ without infective changes in lung fields
– Tuberculosis (Fig. 6.10)	Lymphocytes	
– Sarcoidosis	Macrophages, multinucleated giant cells and T-lymphocytes	CT features of non-caseating granulomas, and classical bilateral hilar adenopathy
– Castleman's disease [10] (Fig. 6.11)	Lymphoid proliferation	Mimics lymphoma, only histopathology can help in differentiation
– Post-transplant nonspecific adenopathy [11]	Lymphocytes (immune-stimulation)	Subcentimetre sized nodes are seen with low grade uptake, which are new, however there is often response seen at the known sites of involvement

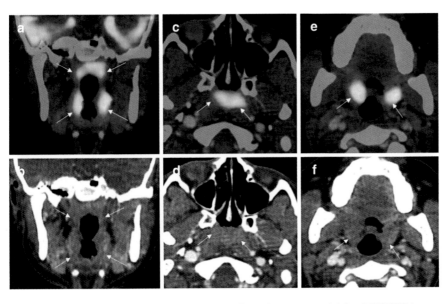

Fig. 6.2 There is bilateral symmetrical intense FDG uptake seen on axial fused PET/CT (**c, e**— arrows) and CT (**d, f**—arrows) images in the region of pharyngeal (**c**) and palatine (**e**) tonsils, seen as ring-like uptake on coronal fused PET/CT (**a**—arrow) and CT (**b**—arrows) images. This uptake is seen in the Waldeyer's ring in the lymphoid tissue

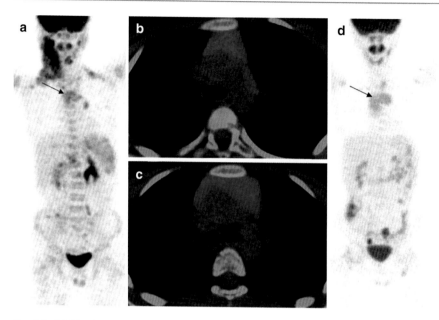

Fig. 6.3 Midline inverted V shaped uptake seen on MIP (**a**—arrow), corresponding to thymic tissue in anterior mediastinum on axial fused PET/CT (**b**—arrow), post4 cycles of chemotherapy, it shows further increase in intensity on MIP (**d**—arrow), seen as rebound thymic hyperplasia (**c**—arrow) on axial fused PET/CT image

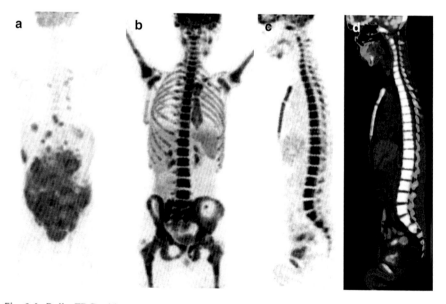

Fig. 6.4 Bulky FDG avid mesenteric mass and liver lesions seen on MIP image (**a**) which received 6 cycles of chemotherapy. Interim PET/CT showed after 4 cycles showed diffuse FDG uptake in axial and appendicular skeleton on coronal and sagittal (MIP, **b** and **c**) and fused PET/CT (**d**) images

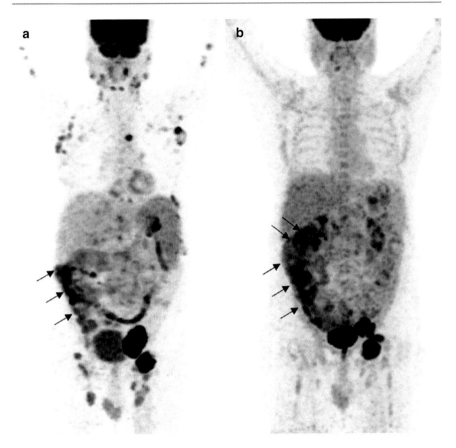

Fig. 6.5 MIP images pre- (**a**) and post-chemotherapy (**b**) show persistent pattern (arrows) of physiological colonic diffuse uptake. Since the nodal disease seen on baseline PET has resolved, the persistent gut uptake is physiological in nature

6.4   Conclusion

FDG PET/CT is the modality of choice for diagnosis, staging and treatment response assessment of lymphomas.

Based on intensity of FDG uptake, lymphomas are classified into high and low grade FDG avid.

Common biochemical pathways of certain physiological and pathological processes lead to variants and pitfalls, which pose significant diagnostic challenges in scan interpretation.

Pattern recognition and accurate interpretation of CT findings can help in overcoming the imaging dilemmas.

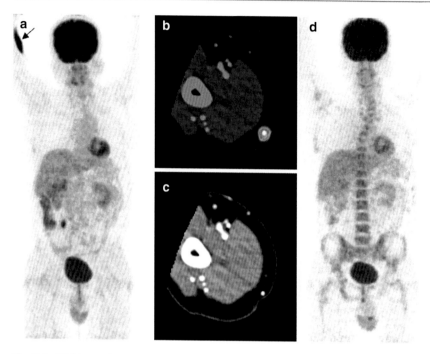

Fig. 6.6 MIP image (**a**—arrow) shows intense FDG uptake at the antecubital injection site confirmed on axial PET/CT (**b**) ad CT (**c**) images, since majority of the tracer had extravasated, the scan was repeated after a day, which shows no uptake at injection site (**d**)

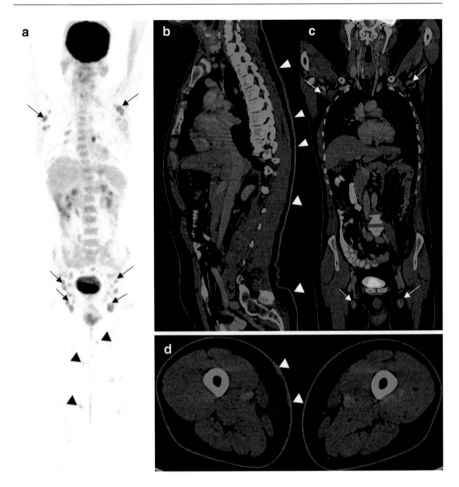

Fig. 6.7 Low grade FDG uptake seen in bilateral axillae and inguinal (**a**—arrows), and in cutaneous regions in medial right thigh (arrow heads). This corresponded to subcentimetre sized bilateral axillary and inguinal nodes (**c**—arrows). Additionally, low grade uptake was seen in cutaneous lesions in the back (**b**—arrowheads) and medial aspect of right thigh (**d**—arrow heads)

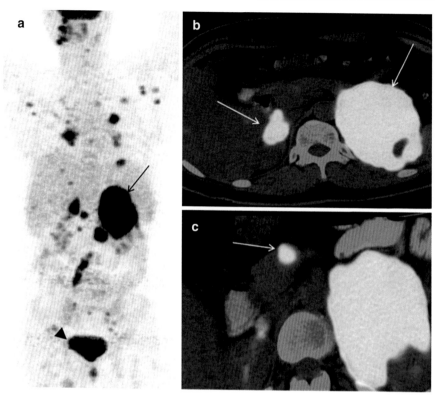

Fig. 6.8 FDG avid lesions seen in bilateral lung, abdomen and retroperitoneal regions (MIP-a), corresponding to bilateral kidney and adrenals (b, c—arrows) suggestive of primary extranodal lymphoma

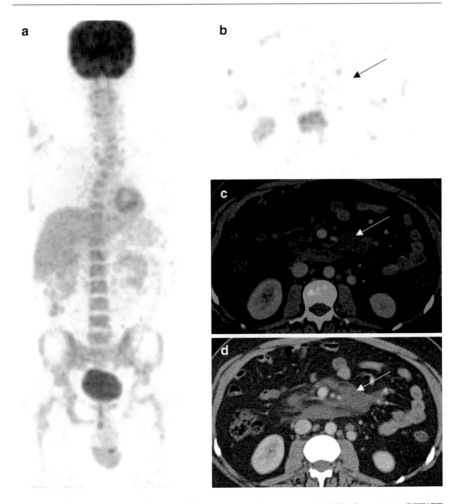

Fig. 6.9 MIP shows no significant FDG uptake (**a**), however, axial PET (**b**—arrow), PET/CT (**c**—arrow) and CT (arrow—**c**) images show localised ill-defined soft tissue with patchy low grade FDG uptake in the mesenteric region suggestive of mesenteric panniculitis, which is an unusual manifestation of lymphoma

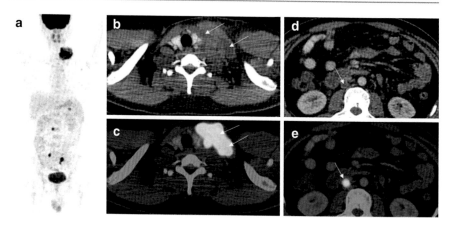

Fig. 6.10 45-year-old male presented with fever, neck swelling and weight loss since 2 months, PET/CT was advised. MIP image shows FDG uptake in left upper thorax and in midline in abdomen and pelvis (**a**). This corresponds to large FDG avid necrotic mass in left supraclavicular region on axial CT (**b**-arrows) and PET/CT (**c**-arrows) images. Also seen is a FDG avid necrotic node (**d**, **e**-arrow) in retrocaval region. Though the pattern was suspicious for lymphomatous involvement, however biopsy was suggestive of granulomatous aetiology

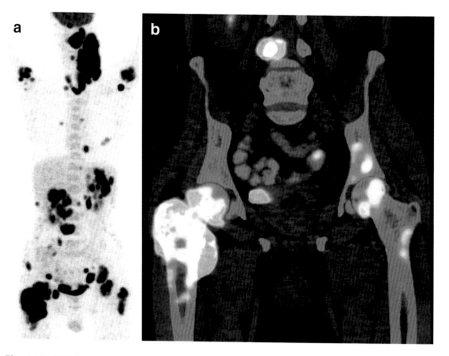

Fig. 6.11 MIP image shows very high grade FDG uptake in neck abdomen and lower extremities (**a**), which corresponded to extensive cervical conglomerated nodes, axillary and mesenteric nodes, and multiple bilateral FDG avid marrow lesions in bilateral pelvic bones and femorii (**b**), this was suspicious for lymphomatous involvement based on PET/CT findings. However, biopsy was suggestive of Castleman's disease, which was a mimic of lymphoma

References

1. Shim HK, Lee WW, Park SY, Kim H, Kim SE. Relationship between FDG uptake and expressions of glucose transporter type 1, type 3, and hexokinase-II in Reed-Sternberg cells of Hodgkin lymphoma. Oncol Res. 2009;17(7):331–7.
2. Cheson BD, Pfistner B, Juweid ME, Gascoyne RD, Specht L, Horning SJ, Coiffier B, Fisher RI, Hagenbeek A, Zucca E, Rosen ST, Stroobants S, Lister TA, Hoppe RT, Dreyling M, Tobinai K, Vose JM, Connors JM, Federico M, Diehl V, International Harmonization Project on Lymphoma. Revised response criteria for malignant lymphoma. J Clin Oncol. 2007;25(5):579–86.
3. McCarten KM, Nadel HR, Shulkin BL, Cho SY. Imaging for diagnosis, staging and response assessment of Hodgkin lymphoma and non-Hodgkin lymphoma. Pediatr Radiol. 2019;49(11):1545–64.
4. Wiyaporn K, Tocharoenchai C, Pusuwan P, Ekjeen T, Leaungwutiwong S, Thanyarak S. Factors affecting standardized uptake value (SUV) of positron emission tomography (PET) imaging with 18F-FDG. J Med Assoc Thai. 2010;93(1):108–14.
5. EsenAkkas B, Gökaslan D, Güner L, IlginKarabacak N. FDG uptake in brown adipose tissue-a brief report on brown fat with FDG uptake mechanisms and quantitative analysis using dual-time-point FDG PET/CT. Rev Esp Med Nucl. 2011;30(1):14–8.
6. Tamayo P, Martín A, Díaz L, Cabrero M, García R, García-Talavera P, Caballero D. 18F-FDG PET/CT in the clinical management of patients with lymphoma. Rev Esp Med NuclImagen Mol. 2017;36(5):312–21.
7. Albano D, Laudicella R, Ferro P, Allocca M, Abenavoli E, Buschiazzo A, Castellino A, Chiaravalloti A, Cuccaro A, Cuppari L, Durmo R, Evangelista L, Frantellizzi V, Kovalchuk S, Linguanti F, Santo G, Bauckneht M, Annunziata S, Young Italian Association of Nuclear Medicine. The role of 18F-FDG PET/CT in staging and prognostication of mantle cell lymphoma: an Italian Multicentric Study. Cancers. 2019;11(12):1831.
8. Adams HJA, Nievelstein RAJ, Kwee TC. Prognostic value of interim and end-of-treatment FDG-PET in follicular lymphoma: a systematic review. Ann Hematol. 2016;95(1):11–8.
9. Kung BT, Seraj SM, Zadeh MZ, Rojulpote C, Kothekar E, Ayubcha C, Ng KS, Ng KK, Au-Yong TK, Werner TJ, Zhuang H, Hunt SJ, Hess S, Alavi A. An update on the role of 18F-FDG-PET/CT in major infectious and inflammatory diseases. Am J Nucl Med Mol Imaging. 2019;9(6):255–73.
10. Han EJ, O JH, Jung SE, Park G, Choi BO, Jeon YW, Min GJ, Cho SG. FDG PET/CT findings of castleman disease assessed by histologic subtypes and compared with laboratory findings. Diagnostics. 2020;10(12):998.
11. von Falck C, Maecker B, Schirg E, Boerner AR, Knapp WH, Klein C, Galanski M. Post transplant lymphoproliferative disease in pediatric solid organ transplant patients: a possible role for [18F]-FDG-PET(/CT) in initial staging and therapy monitoring. Eur J Radiol. 2007;63(3):427–35.

Teaching Cases in Lymphoma as Seen Through FDG PET/CT Images

7

Sayak Choudhury and Venkatesh Rangarajan

Contents

7.1 Staging

Case 1. Stage 1

Images a–c show different spectrums of FDG PET/CT findings of stage 1 lymphomas. (a) A 20-year-old woman with single metabolically active enlarged node in left preauricular region (a1, a2), biopsy revealed Burkitt lymphoma. (b) FDG PET/CT of a 60-year-old man with diffuse large B cell lymphoma (DLBCL) shows hypermetabolic left cervical level II and III nodes (b1, b2). (c) A 28-year-old man with DLBCL shows involvement of oropharynx (c1, c2) and hypopharynx.

S. Choudhury
Department of Nuclear Medicine and Molecular Imaging, Tata Memorial Centre Advanced Centre for Treatment, Research and Education in Cancer, Homi Bhabha National Institute, Mumbai, India

V. Rangarajan (✉)
Department of Nuclear Medicine and Molecular Imaging, Tata Memorial Hospital, Homi Bhabha National Institute (HBNI), Mumbai, India

Teaching Point:
Stage 1 NHL can constitute one single node (a1, a2), single group of nodes (b1, b2) or single extranodal site of involvement (c1, c2).

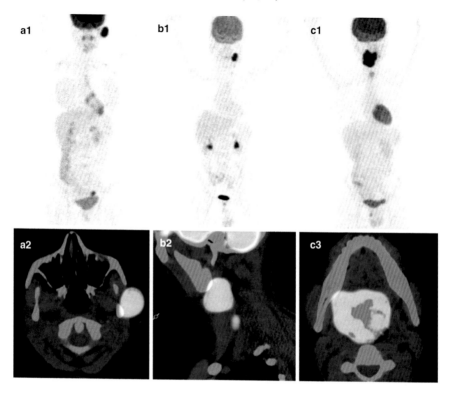

Case 2. Stage 2
F18 FDG PET/CT of a 62-year-old female patient with DLBCL shows hypermetabolic bilateral cervical (arrows in images a and b) and axillary nodes (arrow heads in images a and c) (4 nodal groups on the same side of diaphragm), indicating stage 2 disease.

Teaching Point:
Stage 2 constitutes more than 1 group of nodes on the same side of diaphragm with or without contiguous extranodal involvement.

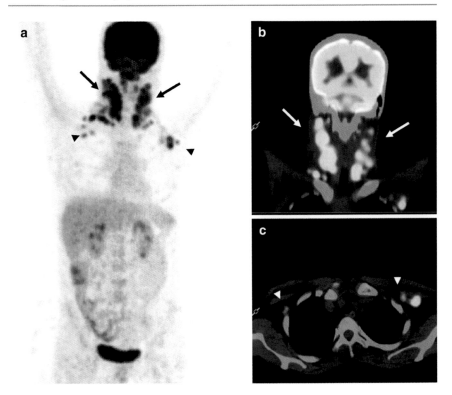

Case 3. Stage 3

FDG PET/CT done in a 31-year-old woman with grade 2 follicular lymphoma, MIP (image a) and fused images (b, c) shows hypermetabolic supradiaphragmatic (left supraclavicular, arrow in image a) and infradiaphragmatic (abdomino-pelvic) lymph nodes (arrow heads in image a).

Teaching Point:

Stage 3 constitutes groups of lymph nodes on both sides of the diaphragm or supradiaphragmatic nodes and involved spleen.

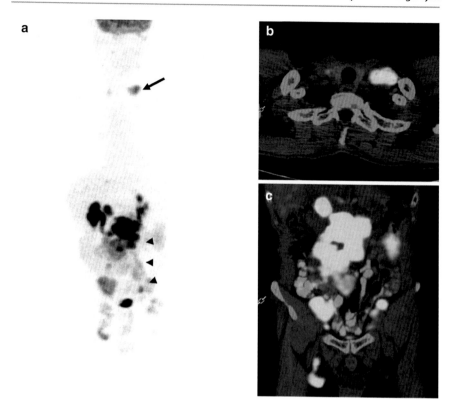

Case 4. Stage 4

In a 74-year-old DLBCL patient staging FDG PET/CT shows metabolically active bilateral cervical, right axillary and mediastinal nodes (arrows in images a–c), metabolically active splenic nodules (arrow heads in images a and d) and hypermetabolic thyroid deposits (notched arrow in images a and b) (extranodal involvement) indicating a stage 4 disease.

Teaching Point:

Stage 4 constitutes nodal involvement with non-contiguous sites of extranodal involvement.

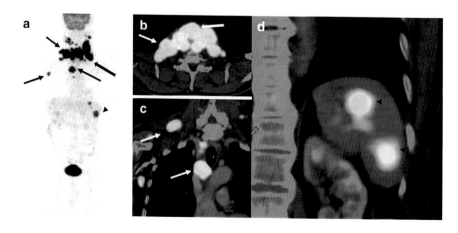

7.2   Spectrum of Marrow Involvement Seen in FDG PET/CT

Case 5. Focal Intense Marrow Uptake
Staging FDG PET/CT in a case of DLBC shows focal intense marrow uptake in left proximal humerus indicating lymphomatous deposit (arrows in images a–c).
   Teaching Point:
   Intense focal FDG uptake in a skeletal site without any obvious cortical changes seen in CT scan is the surest sign of focal marrow involvement by lymphoma.

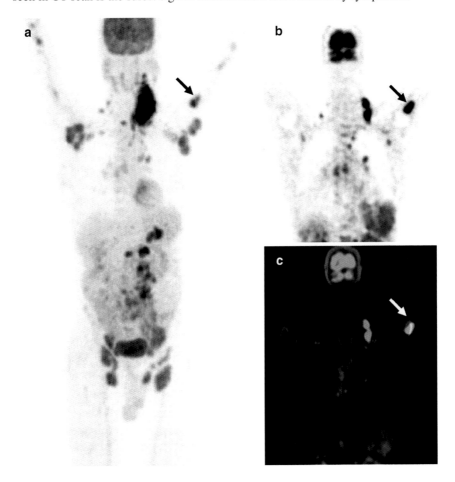

Case 6. Focal Patchy Marrow Uptake
FDG PET/CT in a 50-year-old DLBCL patient shows patchy tracer concentration in visualized marrow indicating lymphomatous involvement. Patchy tracer concentration noted in right ribs, left scapula (arrows in image a), sternum (arrow heads in images a and d) and B/L ilium (notched arrows in images b and c).
   Teaching Point:
   Lymphomatous marrow involvement can be seen as areas of patchy relatively low grade tracer concentration involving various skeletal sites. Key feature is asymmetric distribution of tracer.

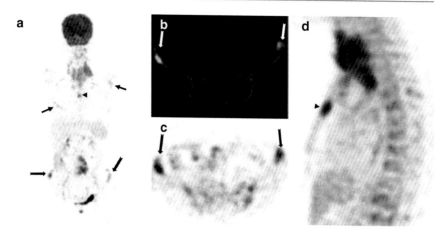

Case 7. Diffuse Patchy Marrow Uptake

FDG PET/CT in a DLBCL patient showing diffusely patchy marrow uptake indicating lymphomatous involvement.

Teaching Point:

Key feature in these types of marrow involvement is patches of increased FDG uptake (black arrow in image b) in a background of diffuse activity. Uptake pattern here is mostly symmetrical.

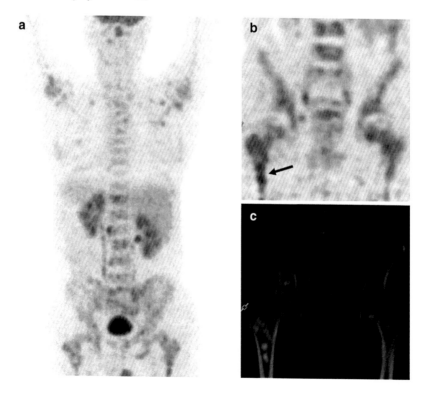

Case 8. Diffuse Symmetrical Continuous Marrow Uptake

FDG PET/CT done in a patient of DLBCL shows diffusely increased marrow metabolism involving the entire visualized skeletal system (image a). Biopsy confirmed lymphomatous marrow involvement.

Teaching Point:

This is the most uncommon pattern of marrow involvement in PET/CT and is often hard to distinguish from reactive marrow stimulation. However, in cases of lymphomatous marrow involvement the uptake is usually higher than that of liver, which is usually not the case for reactive stimulation. Here it is worth noting that diffuse symmetrical low grade marrow metabolism (uptake less than liver) in a high grade FDG avid NHL almost always represents uninvolved marrow. However, FDG PET/CT may miss low volume marrow involvement (10–20% involvement) even in high grade lymphoma such as DLBCL, so a negative PET scan should be corroborated with bone marrow biopsy.

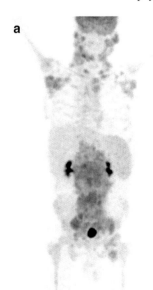
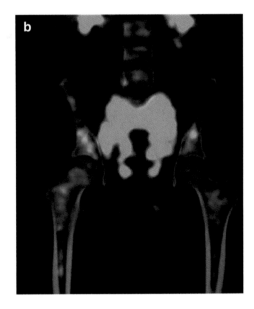

7.3   FDG PET/CT in Assessment of Response to Therapy

Case 9. Deauville Score 1

A stage 2 DLBCL (representative MIP and fused images of staging FDG PET/CT shown in a1, a2) patient after 4 cycles of R-CHOP chemotherapy interim PET (images b1, b2) shows complete disappearance of metabolically active lymphomatous cervical nodes indicating a Deauville's 1 response.

Teaching Point:

Score 1 suggests absence of any discernable FDG uptake.

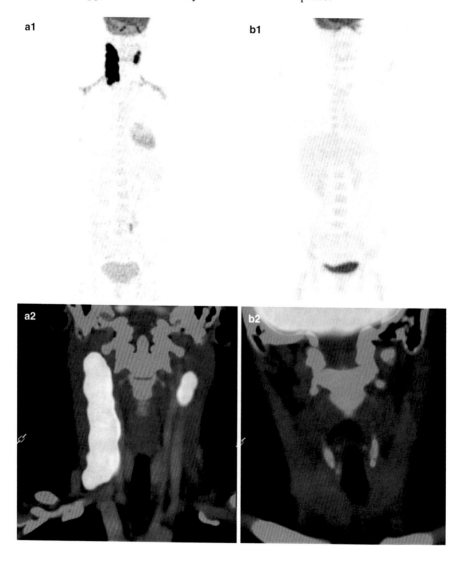

Case 10. Deauville Score 2

In a grade 3 follicular lymphoma patient staging PET/CT showed hypermetabolic supra- and infradiaphragmatic adenopathy along with splenic involvement (images a1, a2, a3). The interim scan after 4 cycles of R-CHOP chemotherapy showed near complete disappearance of hypermetabolic disease, with residual retroperitoneal nodal tissue showing very low grade tracer concentration (arrows in images b2 and b3) which is more than background but equivalent to mediastinum indicating a Deauville's 2 response.

Teaching Point:

Score 2 suggests low grade uptake that is less than or equal to mediastinal blood pool uptake.

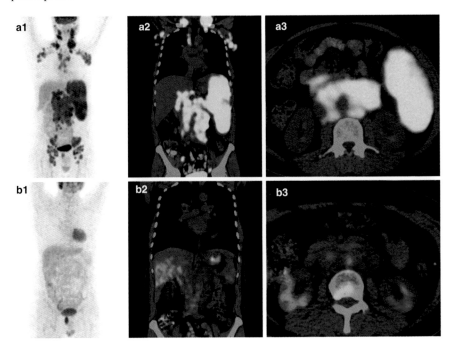

Case 11. Deauville Score 3

A case of relapsed follicular lymphoma (hypermetabolic left inguinal node in image a1 and a2) was treated with second line chemotherapy. After 4 cycles of chemotherapy interim response assessment scan shows low grade uptake in residual left inguinal node (arrows in images b1 and b2).

Teaching Point:

Score 3 suggests uptake more than mediastinum and less than or equal to liver. Scores 1, 2 and 3 consist of complete metabolic response. It should be noted that the Deauville scale should ideally be assessed in the MIP images. The scores are not based on standardized uptake values (SUV) but only on visual grading.

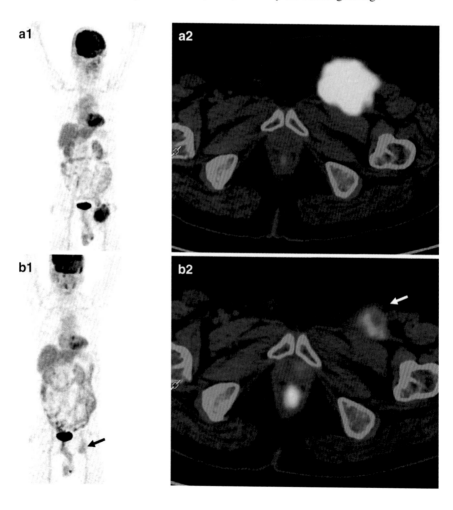

Case 12. Deauville Score 4

FDG PET/CT in a 79-year-old female with DLBCL shows hypermetabolic lesion in right upper GBS and mediastinal nodes (images a1, a2). Interim PET/CT (images b1, b2) done after 4 cycles of R-CHOP chemotherapy shows complete metabolic response in mediastinal nodes with persistent residual disease in right upper alveolus having an uptake of marginally more than liver (arrows in images b1 and b2).

Teaching Point:

Uptake slightly more than liver is considered Deauville score 4. Deauville score of 4 and 5 with decreasing intensity compared to baseline FDG/PET CT is considered partial response.

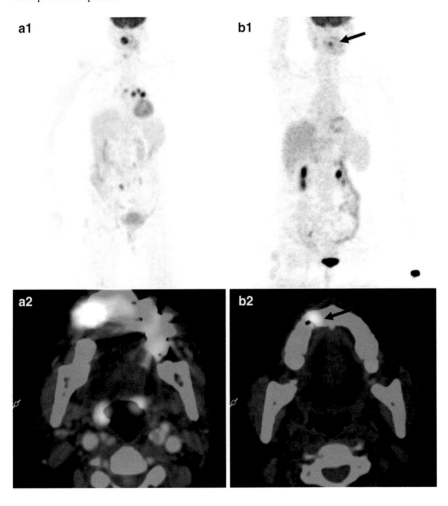

Case 13. Deauville Score 5

A 43-year-old patient suffering from DLBCL, interim PET scan done after 4# chemotherapy (representative images a1–a3), shows significant residual disease in right cervical region. Scan done after completion of 6 cycles of chemotherapy (representative images b1–b3) shows increase in metabolism and size of right cervical nodal mass indicating a Deauville's 5 score and disease progression.

Teaching Point:

Uptake markedly more than liver is considered Deauville score 5.

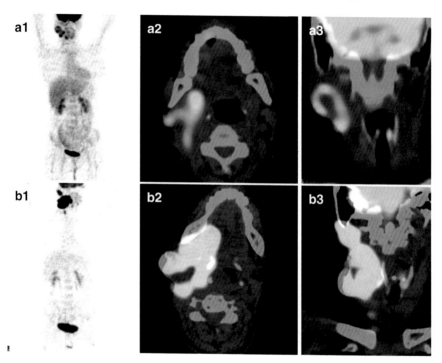

Case 14. Deauville Score 5 (New Lesion)

Relapsed DLBCL on chemotherapy, pre-chemotherapy FDG PET/CT (representative images a1 and a2) showed metabolically active left axillary and retroperitoneal adenopathy (thin arrows in image a1). After 3# of chemotherapy, interim PET/CT (images b1 and b2) shows new metabolically active cervical, mediastinal and retroperitoneal nodes (thin arrows in image b1), indicating Deauville's 5 score and progressive disease.

Teaching Point:

Appearance of new lesion is also considered Deauville 5 score. A Deauville score of 4 to 5 with increasing intensity compared to baseline or any interim scan and/or appearance of new lesion is considered as disease progression.

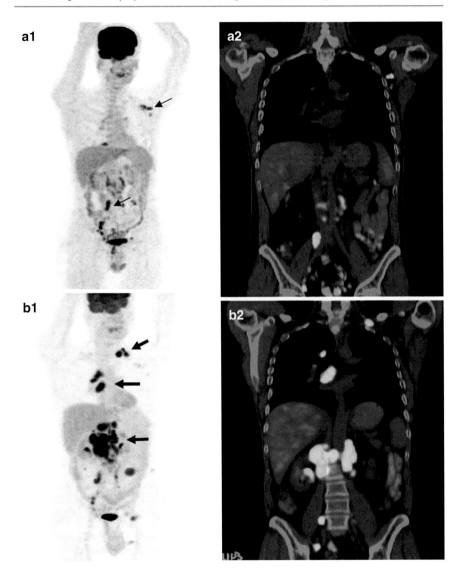

7.4   FDG PET/CT in Transformed Lymphoma

Case 15 A 75-year-old man with follicular lymphoma presented with increase in right inguinal pain and swelling. Biopsy from inguinal lymph node suggested transformation into DLBCL in the background of stage 3B follicular lymphoma. PET/CT scan shows intensely FDG avid retroperitoneal (black arrow in image a and white arrow in image d), right pelvic and B/L inguinal adenopathy (black arrow heads in image a and white arrow head in image e), indicating possible areas of transformation. Relatively low grade FDG uptake noted in cervical, B/L axillary and mediastinal nodes (black and white notched arrows) indicating areas of follicular lymphoma that are not showing transformation.

Teaching Point:

Indolent low grade lymphomas may undergo histologic transformation into aggressive, high grade lymphomas. Transformation commonly occurs to DLBCL, less commonly to other types of high grade lymphoma, including Burkitt and T cell/histiocyte-rich B cell lymphoma (TCRBCL). Diagnosing transformation is crucial since management of indolent lymphomas and transformed high grade lymphomas are completely different and transformed lymphomas typically have worse prognosis. FDG PET/CT can help identifying the ideal site for biopsy to detect nodal/extranodal transformation.

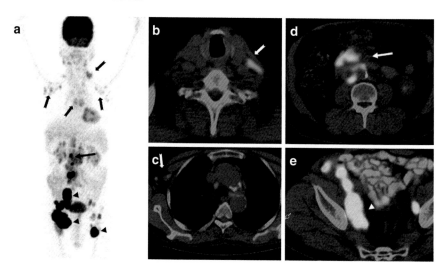

7.5 Extranodal Site Involvement Seen in FDG PET/CT

Case 16. Bowel Involvement in Lymphoma

Burkitt lymphoma in a 11-year-old child who presented with abdominal distention and pain. MIP image (a) and fused image (c) show metabolically active lesion involving mediastinum and abdomen. Abdominal soft tissue noted involving the small bowel loops and adjacent peritoneum. Some of the bowel loops show aneurysmal dilatation (black arrows in image b).

Teaching Point:
Aneurysmal dilatation of bowel may be seen in B cell small bowel lymphomas due to replacement of muscularis propria and destruction of autonomic nervous system by lymphoma.

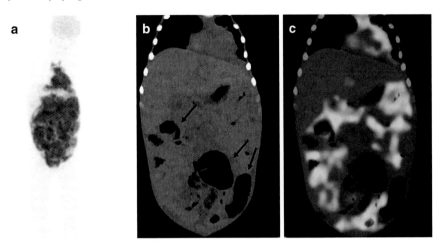

Case 17 Primary Gastric Lymphoma
High grade NHL (grey zone between Burkitt lymphoma and CD10 positive DLBCL) in a 28-year-old man who presented with abdominal pain. PET/CT shows hypermetabolic diffuse circumferential wall thickening involving distal body, antrum and pylorus of stomach (arrow in image b).

Teaching Point:
Gastric lymphoma is characterized by marked thickening of stomach wall. Stomach lymphoma is the most common site of extranodal involvement in NHL. Most common histopathological subtypes of primary gastric lymphoma are DLBCL with or without mucosa-associated lymphoid tissue (MALT) component and MALT lymphoma of the marginal zone.

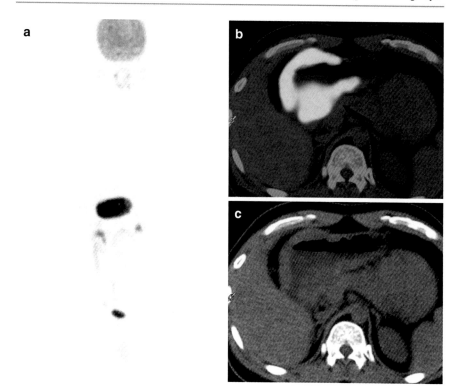

Case 18. Primary Bone Lymphomas

(a) T cell/histiocyte-rich large B cell lymphoma presented with left femur lesion. FDG PET/CT (images a1–a4) shows hypermetabolic permeative lytic lesion involving distal epimetadiaphysis of left femur with significant extramedullary soft tissue and periosteal reaction (image a3). Pathological fracture also noted (image a3). Metabolically active left external iliac nodes (black arrows in image A4). (b) High grade B cell lymphoma(DLBCL) presented with lytic expansile lesion involving right proximal humerus (images b1–b3). No extraosseous involvement seen.

Teaching Point:

Primary bone lymphoma is a rare entity (<5% of all primary bone tumours and <1% of all NHL). For a bone malignancy to be called a primary bone lymphoma there should be histopathological documentation of lymphoma in a solitary (or multi focal) bone lesion without any documented nodal involvement (except regional lymph nodes). Most common morphology in CT/ radiograph is permeative lysis with wide zone of transition. Most common sites of involvement are long bones (femur>humerus>tibia). DLBCL is the most common histology.

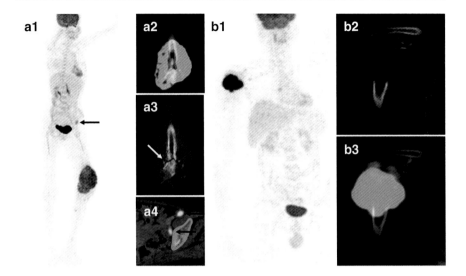

Case 19. Renal Involvement in Lymphoma

A 30-year-old male with lymphoblastic lymphoma presented with pain and swelling in right inguinal region. FDG PET/CT shows hypermetabolic lytic lesion involving right pelvis (arrowhead in image a), and bilateral bulky kidneys with hypermetabolic hypoenhancing deposits replacing normal renal parenchyma (black arrow in image b).

Teaching Point:

Renal lymphoma is usually part of multisystemic lymphoma. The common presentations seen in PET/CT are (a) multiple FDG avid masses/deposits involving both kidneys coupled with enlarged metabolically active retroperitoneal nodes, (b) direct invasion from retroperitoneal adenopathy, (c) solitary hypermetabolic mass usually homogeneous hypodense as compared to the enhancing renal cortex, (d) diffuse hypermetabolic cortical infiltration. Frequently bilateral involvement is seen. Renal lymphomas show intense FDG uptake, to differentiate from urine activity PET scan after intravenous frusemide injection may be helpful.

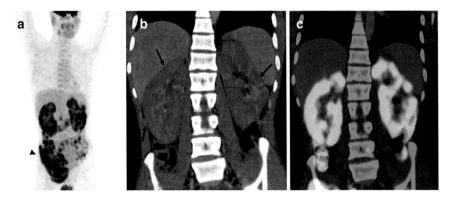

Case 20. Cutaneous T Cell Lymphoma

FDG PET/CT in a 60-year-old patient with cutaneous T cell lymphoma shows an FDG avid large ulcerated skin lesion along the medial aspect of left thigh (thin arrows in images a–c) along with multiple smaller nodular cutaneous plaques in right thigh and B/L calf regions (thin arrows in images a, d and e). FDG avid left inguinal node is also seen (thick arrows in images a–c).

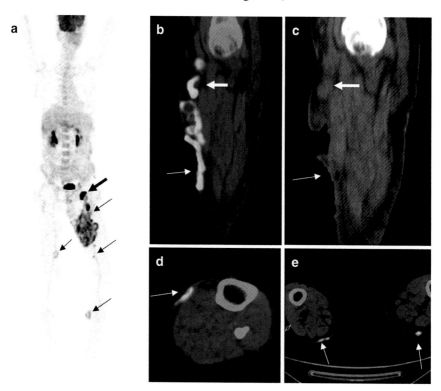

Case 21. Subcutaneous Panniculitis-like T Cell Lymphoma (A Rare Form of Peripheral T Cell Lymphoma Presents with Panniculitis)

A 41-year-old man with relapsed subcutaneous panniculitis-like T cell lymphoma. F18 FDG PET/CT shows multiple areas of subcutaneous soft tissue stranding, nodules, mesenteric stranding and nodules, and liver lesion. Increased FDG uptake noted in diffuse subcutaneous stranding involving B/L legs and the shin area (white arrows in images b and c). Hypermetabolic ground glassing and fat stranding noted involving mesentery (black arrows in images d and e). FDG avid nodule noted in subcutaneous plane of anterior abdominal wall (white notched arrows in images f and g). Focal FDG avid liver lesion seen (arrow head in image h).

Teaching Points:

1. Cutaneous T cell lymphomas may present with patches, plaques or erythroderma which may be difficult to appreciate in conventional CT scan. However, PET scan usually shows uptake and can help detect the smaller cutaneous plaques. Non-attenuation corrected (NAC) PET image may help in detecting superficial cutaneous lesions with low grade uptake. To detect areas of extracutaneous involvement FDG PET/CT is crucial.
2. Subcutaneous panniculitis-like T cell lymphoma is a rare disorder and may systemically present as inflammatory panniculitis. PET/CT findings are usually metabolically active nodular lesions in the subcutaneous fat plane or diffuse ground glass opacity and fat stranding. FDG PET/CT may help identify areas of visceral, nodal, marrow involvement.

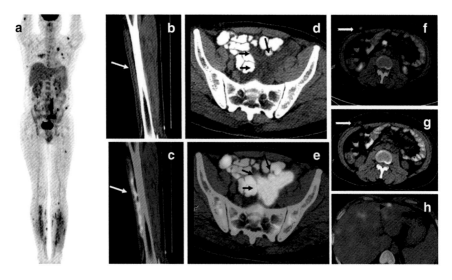

Case 22. CNS Involvement in Lymphoma

(a) A 45-year-old man with primary CNS lymphoma, PET/CT (images a1–a3) showed hypermetabolic homogeneously enhancing solid periventricular space occupying lesion in right basal ganglia region(white arrows in images a2 and a3). (b) A 46-year-old patient presented with giddiness and imbalance while walking. MRI suggested left cerebellar hemisphere lesion causing obstructive hydrocephalous, patient underwent sub-occipital craniotomy (images b2, b3). Histopathology showed high grade NHL. PET/CT (images b1–b5) shows focal FDG avid marrow lesions in sacrum and left ischio-pubic ramus (bold arrows in images b1, b4 and b5), indicating extra cranial lymphomatous disease. (c) A 50-year-old male with lymphoblastic lymphoma with secondary CNS involvement. PET/CT (images c1–c6) shows FDG avid homogenously enhancing solid lesion in right frontal lobe near the cortex (images c2 and c4), FDG avid enhancing thickened B/L trigeminal nerve trunk seen traversing the B/L cavernous sinus region (arrow heads in images c4 and c5) and FDG avid mediastinal adenopathy (image c6).

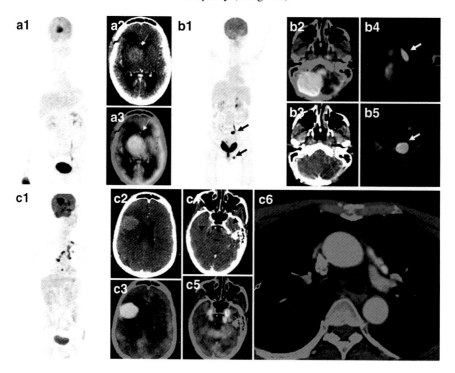

Case 23. Leptomeningeal Involvement in Lymphoma

Secondary leptomeningeal involvement in a case of relapsed T cell rich B cell lymphoma. FDG PET/CT shows diffuse leptomeningeal FDG uptake noted along brain and spinal cord up to D10 vertebral level suggesting lymphomatous involvement (arrows in images a–c). FDG avid right axillary and mediastinal nodes also noted (notched arrows in image d).

Teaching Point:

1. Typical appearance of a primary CNS lymphoma in FDG PET/CT is an intensely FDG avid homogeneously enhancing hyperdense well defined solid space occupying lesion. May present as single mass or multiple masses. Typical location is often supratentorial usually in contact with the subarachnoid/ependymal surfaces like the periventricular region. Usually haemorrhage and necrosis not seen and they may cross corpus callosum. However, this appearance is typical in a non-immunocompromised patient. In immunocompromised patients, the appearance may be a lot heterogeneous, featuring central non-enhancement/necrosis and less likely haemorrhage.

2. Multi-parametric MRI is the diagnostic modality of choice. However, FDG PET/CT helps in locating extracranial sites of disease and rules out secondary CNS involvement in a case of systemic lymphoma.
3. Leptomeningeal involvement if present is usually secondary and is generally part of systemic lymphoma. Primary CNS lymphoma may rarely show leptomeningeal involvement.

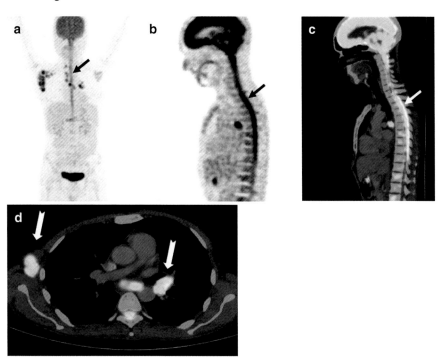

Case 24. Neurolymphomatosis

(1) PET/CT (images a1–a7) in a patient with relapsed cutaneous T cell lymphoma showed increased FDG uptake involving the thickened left tibial nerve soon after its origin at the apex of popliteal fossa (thin arrows in images a1, a2, a4 and a6). FDG avid thickening also noted in the thickened right deep fibular (peroneal nerve) along the anterior compartment of right leg (thick arrows in images a3, a5 and a7). The fusiform thickening of the nerve trunk is seen as an area of homogenous soft tissue density without any intervening fat spaces unlike the surrounding muscles which show intermuscular fat spaces between muscle fibres (image a3). (2) A 57-year-old disseminated mantel cell lymphoma. FDG PET/CT (images b1–b5) shows linear FDG uptake along the course of bilateral sciatic nerves (notched arrows).

Teaching Point:

Neurolymphomatosis (NL) is a rare extranodal manifestation of non-Hodgkin lymphoma characterized by direct infiltration of malignant lymphoma cells into the peripheral nerves. Peripheral nerve involvement in FDG PET/CT is usually seen as uptake along the nerve trunk, the nerve may also be thickened.

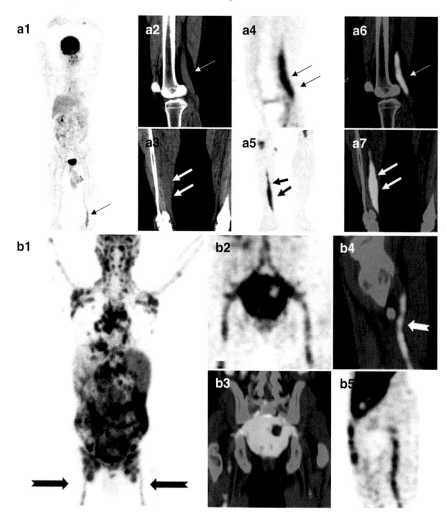